The Food Allergy Plan

D1147700

KEITH MUMBY, MB ChB

A working physician's practical and tested method

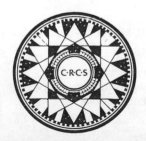

CRCS PUBLICATIONS
P.O. Box 20850
Reno, NV 89515
U.S.A.

Publishers Note: This book does not attempt to diagnose or treat specific illnesses. It is advisable to seek professional advice or to consult your physician in every case where you are in doubt about your health, particularly when you have persistent pain or any other continuous symptom. The publisher of this book takes no responsibility for the reader's health or use or misuse of the information contained herein.

Library of Congress Cataloging-in-Publication Data

Mumby, Keith.
The food allergy plan.

Originally published: London : Unwin Paperbacks, 1985.
Bibliography: p.
Includes index.
1. Food allergy--Popular works. 2. Food allergy--Diet therapy. I. Title. [DNLM: 1. Diet Therapy--popular works. 2. Food Hypersensitivity--popular works. WD 310 M962f]
RC596.M85   1986   616.97'5   86-14801
ISBN 0-916360-33-4 (pbk.)

FIRST U.S.A. EDITION—Originally published in Great Britain
    by Unwin Paperbacks

INTERNATIONAL STANDARD BOOK NUMBER: 0-916360-33-4

Published in the United States by: CRCS Publications
        Distributed in the United States by
        CRCS Publications

Contents

Acknowledgements

My thanks are due to my dear friends, Ted Hamlyn and Dorothy West, for putting my feet on the road; to Theron Randolph and Richard Mackerness as great pioneers and teachers; and for forbearance, to my wife Pauline, without whose help my busy practice would be impossible to run.

Introduction: The Miracle Eating Plan

If a diet had been discovered which cured a number of serious illnesses including eczema, dermatitis, migraine, colitis, asthma, high blood pressure, obesity, depression, schizophrenia, alcoholism and peptic ulcer plus routinely alleviated a whole host of minor complaints such as abdominal bloating, mouth ulcers, itchy eyes, difficulty waking in the morning, overweight, palpitations, a flu-like state that *isn't flu*, panic attacks, 'foggy brain syndrome' and catarrh, you would rightly call it a miracle diet, wouldn't you? Perhaps you are wondering if such a diet is even possible. Well, it is and it does exist. It has been known to a small group of skilled doctors who call themselves clinical ecologists for a number of years now. It is the subject of this book. I use it regularly in my clinic, and it really can do all that is claimed above. Its concern is with food allergies, and it will uncover those items in *your* diet which may be resulting in non-optimum health.

There is a growing awareness that correct eating and good health go hand in hand. What was not realised until very recently was just to what extent that simple observation is true. With the discovery of the phenomenon of food allergies and the recognition of their widespread harmful effects, the door has been opened for the cure of a wide variety of diseases. It has been estimated that *over half of all illnesses* reported to doctors are caused by food allergies, so this condition is not rare. In addition, there is a great deal of minor symptomatology which is not reported at all: everyone considers it 'normal' to have a few aches and pains. Good health is often taken to be the mere absence of disease. Yet abundant energy, well-being, clarity of thinking and zest should be your lot. If this isn't the case, then the advice in this book probably applies to you.

The Food Allergy Plan is much more than just a diet: it takes you step by step through the unmasking of hidden allergy

1

which may be spoiling your life. What is *revolutionary* about this plan is that it is *not* a fixed diet. We have meat-free, fruit-free, arthritis, slimming and beauty diets galore, but they all share one fundamental flaw: *no one diet can possibly suit every case.* An incorrect diet may make things worse. Society is currently in the grip of what one of my doctor friends called 'fibre fever', yet even this justifiably famous plan actually makes some people worse: wheat allergics have a very bad time eating fibre, which is mostly wheat-derived.

The tracking down and uncovering of the hidden allergy effect has probably been the single most important medical discovery this century, measured simply in terms of the *amount* of human suffering now able to be alleviated. Naturally, public interest is high in this new *safe* approach to healing. Many people who thought they were destined to be ill for life – and perhaps had been *told* so by doctors who should know better – are waking up to the fact that recovery may be attained merely through eating and drinking differently. As with all great discoveries, the essence of this breakthrough is that it is simple; yet the implications are far-reaching. Once the basic principles are grasped, a whole host of apparently complicated and seemingly unrelated phenomena begin to make sense. In a way, this book and others like it become maps and compasses for an adventure of exploration: you can sail out onto unknown seas of knowledge, make discoveries for yourself, chart new localities and all the time know where you are, what is happening and why.

Unfortunately, the medical profession as a whole is entrenched in the belief that diet is unimportant, despite the fact that Hippocrates over two thousand years ago stated that no healing could be truly successful without attention being paid to what the patient was eating. Instead, the conventional doctor blunders on, with newer and more dangerous drugs, always ready with the knife, spurred on by more and more obscure laboratory 'investigations' until the patient is lost in a welter of science. One wonders where it will all end, for whereas in any other profession a narrowness of view is nothing more than an infantile and unbecoming failure, in medicine it is a dangerous, almost criminal, neglect of duty from which only the patient suffers. A doctor has a certain responsibility to do the best for his or her patient, and that means keeping abreast of any area of new knowledge which may help. Sadly, the history of medicine does not reflect this responsibility: the first users of anaesthetics were struck off as frauds; Dr Semmelweis of Vienna was scorned to the point of suicide for suggesting that doctors wash their hands before examining women in childbed; and, nearer our own period, pencillin – arguably the greatest drug of all time – was ignored as a discovery when it could have saved *millions* of lives. Even today, homoeopathy, which cures gently by taking into account the whole person as opposed to merely a part, is fought against with blind fury by doctors who have never prescribed any of its remedies.

You may think I write bitterly about the resistance of medical practitioners to accept this new work – and you are right, of course. I have had my share of scorn and ridicule from colleagues who have never once taken the trouble to visit my clinic and see if the work I do is really valid. Yet what I have experienced is as nothing compared to what the great pioneers of this field in America and here in the United Kingdom have had to endure – my hat is off to them. But what concerns me most is the disparagement and abuse that patients themselves sometimes have to undergo because of their allergies. So many times I have had before me sad and dispirited human beings who break into tears of relief when they realise that someone, at last, is willing to listen to their problems and *believe* them. As a rule they have been scolded or told they were neurotic and 'imagining' things. Many of them feel they are a burden to their family doctor when, in some cases, the opposite seems to be true.

I know from the fact that every time I speak on the radio or one of our cases is featured in the press we are deluged with calls for help that very many people are anxious for help and *don't know where to get it.* That is how this book came to be written. If your own doctor refuses to help, there is little you can do except try to sort things out for yourself. Perhaps this do-it-yourself volume will enable you to do just that. I should like to think that many of you will succeed with its guidance. It will be pleasant to know that I may make some new friends even if I never meet them!

Confronted with the wonder of what remission of pain and misery is possible, I feel rather overawed; and until this feeling deserts me I shall go on giving my best, because never before have I so enjoyed my career or felt so proud to be a healer. I make no claims to discoveries in the field of allergies, but the method which follows is my own and is offered freely to whoever is in need of it.

Within weeks – or even days – you could be free of a chronic or lifelong affliction. Without exaggeration, the lame can walk again, the respiratory cripple can breathe, the sickly and weak become strong, pain and misery diminish to but a memory. It really is a miracle: hundreds of thousands of cases from all over the world attest to it. I am very proud to bring you the Food Allergy Plan.

1

Cases, Cases, Cases . . .

This book contains new and exciting revelations about diet and how the avoidance of harmful or hostile foods can help those who are not in optimum health (almost everybody!). A small but rapidly growing band of doctors have been showing that a tremendous amount of human illness and suffering can be attributed to the fact that foods can make you ill. This is a startling idea, so much so that many in the medical profession have difficulty in accepting it. But you must judge for yourself, and I hope the picture as it unfolds plus the chance to try out the techniques will enable you to rise above popular prejudice and opinion and enter the realm of true discovery.

To give you some idea of what it can achieve, here are some case histories from my clinical notebooks. These are not even the most sensational recoveries I know of. The ones included here are typical of a wide variety of conditions and are chosen because they show ordinary people with ordinary, though in some cases severe, diseases – the kind you might be suffering from. These are not medical reports of the kind that I would supply to a fellow medical practitioner, just plain stories, told in everyday English that illustrate the point. The scientific and technical basis of these recoveries are fully covered later in the book. Each case was put through the Food Allergy Plan exactly as given, and the results are summarised. Long before the final chapter you should be able to achieve the same success for yourself. The trick is to work out what your own *personal ideal diet* is.

It cannot be stressed enough that there is no such thing as a universal health diet: what suits some people will make others ill. This fact has been glossed over by all previous writers on this topic. In that sense, this is a revolutionary programme. Although the basic discoveries of food allergies were not made by me, this plan is my own, worked out over many years of treating patients. These ideas are not theoretical but intensely practical, the techniques I myself use every day in my clinic, and everything you will read here has been tried and tested thousands of times. It is a *working* system, and as such it has a great deal to commend it.

Many people – especially doctors, remain sceptical or indifferent to these vital new discoveries. That does not mean that the information given here is not of concern to *you*. The only way you will know for sure, as with many interesting new ideas and schemes, is to try it out for yourself. So for you it is a true voyage of discovery: the maps are there and the route all worked out, but one aspect remains a mystery and that is *you the person*. I have no idea in advance what you will discover about your health and eating habits; I only know it could be very, very important. The fun of finding out is all yours – I wish you luck.

Case no. 1: Severe arthritis

Mac was a friendly 50-year-old Scot, lively, intelligent and well educated – everything the emigré from north of the border is traditionally noted for. He was hard-working and successful too, one of the army of quiet businessmen of the type who once helped Britain build and maintain her empire across the globe. At the peak of his career he was senior executive in a Far Eastern company, travelling the world and enjoying the respect of colleagues from Manchester to Tokyo. He had earned his status and was entitled to be proud of it.

Then arthritis struck. At first it was no more than an uncomfortable periodic ache, but unfortunately it soon progressed and began to worsen with relentless speed. Within a few years he was a very sick man and his way of life had become very restricted. The pain was severe, but the main enemy was stiffness: some days it would take him one-and-a-half hours to get out of bed and get moving sufficiently to leave the house or hotel. Although he tried to conceal his difficulty, it soon became obvious to his workfellows. Instead of enjoying his work as he always had, he suddenly found in it only embarrassment and physical discomfort.

Things drifted for a while. Various doctors treated him, but this amounted to no more than painkillers which did little to help and made no impact on the progress of the disease. Inevitably, it became impossible for him to do his job, energy-consuming and demanding as it was. The final straw came in Japan with a heart attack which was followed by angina – pain due to cardiac underperfusion brought on by exercise. Mac was pensioned off, so to speak, on health grounds and sent home to this country. There he was given work that was much easier, but it was very unfulfilling for someone like him. He felt as if he had been relegated to the back row, and it cast a long, deep shadow on all his achievements and his career as a whole.

By the time he came to my clinic he was an unhappy and frustrated man. His body was causing him great anguish, and his mind had begun to lose the razor-sharp edge to which he had always been accustomed. His speech was broken up by embarrassingly long pauses while he tried to resume his train of thought. It is particularly sad when a condition of this sort brings down the 'big' ones: men and women of great zest and skill, the 'doers' in life that most of us envy. They take it very hard. And to add to his gloom, he had been told by every doctor he had spoken to that his debility was permanent and 'incurable'; they said he would have to 'live with it' (a favourite phrase, and an unbearably depressing one).

From the first I suspected food allergies. High-fliers are often high-livers, and a study of his diet showed this to be the case. I explained to him the Food Allergy Plan (I don't call it that with patients; the correct name is elimination and challenge dieting) and he started on it. To his immense delight, within ten days he noticed an improvement. The pain and swelling in his joints began to subside. He started waking with a clear head and a body that responded within minutes instead of hours. He wasn't of an age to leap out of bed, but in contrast to the way he had been that was how it felt to him. Each day, especially the mornings, again became something to look forward to instead of to dread. On his second visit he looked and felt a new man.

We then set about finding out which foods had been causing the trouble. I allowed him to slowly, one at a time and over a few weeks, reintroduce the foods he had been avoiding. Those which caused a recurrence of his symptoms he was instructed to steer clear of. If there was no reaction, that food was considered safe and allowed to remain in his diet.

In this way we discovered he was allergic to a number of foods but in particular wheat (the worst), chicken and orange. Providing he avoids them he remains happy and reasonably well. It isn't a complete recovery, but enough to allow him to do as he wishes, namely work, travel to the Far East several times a year and generally pick up life where had he left off. As an added bonus, his angina has disappeared: he is off all drugs and is capable of carrying out normal physical activities, even a full round of golf, without pain. Yet if he eats wheat, especially bread, his symptoms return with a vengeance – so much so that he no longer tries to test it and avoids it completely, even in gravy thickening. As he sees it, it simply isn't worth the trouble and pain; it is far easier to eat differently as outlined in this book. A miracle? He thinks so, and I must admit that even after all this time I haven't lost my sense of wonder when someone gets well like that.

Case no. 2: Mysterious swellings

Mrs G was a 47-year-old married social worker. Apart from being a little highly strung, she had enjoyed good health for most of her adult life. She had raised three fine children and was approaching the time of life when she and her husband would be entitled to start looking forward to enjoying the fruits of their labours.

The dream of a comfortable middle age was, however, rudely shattered by sudden ill health: not cancer, high blood pressure, a coronary or any of the well-known sinister and dangerous conditions, yet to her it was frightening and debilitating and it had a hardly less damaging effect on her well-being than possible more serious complaints might have done. About four years before she came to see me, sudden mysterious swellings had started to develop. These were not continually present but came in attacks that occurred every few weeks right out of the blue. There was no pattern to it: there might be several occurrences in a month, or alternatively none for many weeks. Her face was most prominently affected, and when the condition was severe her eyes would close up completely. Sometimes the throat was involved and the swelling would press on the windpipe, making breathing difficult; she would then be forced to tilt her head back in order to get air in and out of her lungs. Naturally, these episodes were quite terrifying. A doctor would be rushed to her for emergency treatment, but there was always the haunting fear that she might suffocate before help arrived.

It was no ordinary puffiness but a huge increase in size: her head would feel almost too heavy to lift because of the great weight of fluid. She looked like a gargoyle, grotesque and unnatural, so much so that her friends could hardly recognise her. Of course, she was quite unable to work for fear of scaring her clients. The protuberances would disappear as mysteriously as they had come, only to return at some point later. Doctors were unable to diagnose the reason or to help. It was no use staying permanently on drugs when there was no way of knowing when the condition would strike next. The attacks were getting to be more frequent, and by the time we met she was depressed and desperate.

My first question was 'When did it start?' She remembered the occasion clearly. It was in a traffic jam, she had been driving her car and had, like most of the other drivers, become steadily more frustrated and overwrought mentally. The fumes had been choking, and the heat (it was a summer's day) had made her feel faint and weary. When the traffic eventually got on the move again she had found herself in tears: perhaps it was due to stress, or to the fact that her eyes felt red and itchy – she wasn't sure. But by the time she got home and looked in the mirror the truth was obvious: some strange and frightening reaction had caused her face to puff up and her eyes to turn bloodshot and sore. After that the problem recurred with increasing frequency. It would be tempting to assume an allergy to traffic fumes, but it is worth noting that she was exposed on a very large number of occasions to equally high concentrations and had no reaction. Furthermore, she would sometimes get this swelling without even going out of doors. Inconsistencies like this are fully explained in this book.

Having drawn up a full history of her case, I found plenty of supportive symptoms such as aching muscles, a general slowing down, insomnia and flu-like attacks (that were not flu), to

suggest allergy, including food allergy, as the cause of the
trouble. So we discussed the plan given in this book and she
decided to give it a try.

To cut the rest of the story short, the treatment was a
complete success. She carried out tests on herself using the
procedure outlined in a later chapter and found it was best to
avoid certain foods: *wheat, corn, chicken,* cheese, egg, milk and
coffee (the items in italics were the worst offenders). Since then
there has been no recurrence of her condition; not only that,
but she feels fitter and healthier than she can remember being in
years. I fully expected to have to delve into chemical allergies,
but this turned out to be unnecessary. Not that this proves she
is not allergic to chemicals; simply that, with her diet under
control, she can cope with these as well as the rest of us can.

Case no. 3: Behavioural problems

The next case is that of a schoolboy which is so like the story of
hundreds and thousands of others that I think it a great shame
that all teachers, as well as parents, are unaware of the
importance of diet in influencing behaviour. Luckily this tale
has a happy ending, but so many do not: often delinquency,
even crime, follows in the wake of poor eating, and the helpless
teachers and mystified parents never suspect the real reason.
Such a pity, when the cure is so easy, as this book shows.

I have allowed the lad's mother to tell the story in the form
of a letter to me:

Dear Dr Mumby,
It's marvellous to be able to write and tell you what a complete
success your dietary programme has been with our son Alan. As
you know, we had some awful problems, but now, thanks to you,
he is the lovely boy he promised to be as a toddler. Let me go
back to the beginning.

Alan as a little baby was always so happy and a delight to be
with. In fact we had no inkling of what was to follow. It wasn't
until he reached the age of about three, when he started to go to
playschool, that things started to go wrong.

We were told that he behaved rather aggressively towards the
other children and that he was demanding and seemed to want
the attention of the group leader all the time. We were surprised,
because this was so untypical. We talked it over and assumed it

was just a phase he was going through and that he needed time to adjust. But in fact it got worse.

Then we suspected that he had communication problems. Although quite bright and certainly not backward for his age, his speech was virtually non-existent. We decided this should be tackled vigorously and, after much cajoling, we managed to get professional help from a succession of speech therapists. This paid off in the sense that his speech is now almost perfect, unlike that of many of his peers. But his behaviour, unfortunately, did not improve.

When he started school we became very worried about his attitude to everything and everybody, his moods seemed to swing from being loving and caring to becoming an uncooperative and introverted little 'monkey' [sic].

Over the next couple of years things got worse and worse. Although we knew for certain that he was bright, he was consistently underachieving in his studies and we were told he was a disruptive influence on the rest of the class. He was always in trouble, he would 'forget' to bring home his homework, and we would get frequent disturbing phone calls from the head-mistress telling us what a problem he was. She had tried many times to admonish or discipline him, but nothing she – or we – said seemed to have any effect.

It wasn't only school that was affected: it began to be noticeable he was being invited out less and less and his friends became fewer. One day we were told by a helpful parent that it was because his moods swung so violently from happy to surly, aggressive and back. It was so unpredictable that it was most disconcerting for others.

Then he began to complain of tummy ache in the mornings. At first we thought this was just a ruse to get out of going to school, but he had it during the holidays also. Headaches began to follow, and we finally started to take him seriously when he told us he was getting pains in his joints, mainly the legs. The doctor said it was nothing to worry about, just 'growing pains', but that didn't seem right to us.

Meanwhile his behaviour was worse than ever. We tried coaxing, smacking, cuddling and penalties over the years, but nothing had any effect. He would do all sorts of strange, destructive things, such as ripping pyjamas, tearing books, smashing up, etc., and when we asked him why he did it he would break down and cry. He had no idea why he was doing it – he certainly didn't want to behave like that – and it was pitiful to watch the conflict going on inside him. We felt so helpless.

Then one day we heard of you and your clinic. We thought

anything was worth a try. Since then we have never looked back. He has reverted to being a normal, sociable young boy, we are free of the tension and worry, and he is so happy and calm it is a pleasure to watch him.

We are not pretending that sticking to the diet has been easy. It is very restrictive for someone his age. But we have explained to Alan that it isn't for ever, maybe just eighteen months or two years. So long as he keeps to it, all is well.

We have begun to reintroduce certain foods, albeit gradually, to his diet. The ones he cannot tolerate are withdrawn again. This way we have a very clear idea of what foods affect him. It seems doubtful if he will ever be able to take eggs in any great amount. When he eats anything with egg in he immediately gets a headache and pains in his chest, stomach and joints. It's a pity – we keep our own hens!

We have had one or two ups and downs. A few weeks ago Alan crept into the kitchen while we were sleeping and demolished half a cake and some biscuits. The following day he was dreadful. All his antisocial mannerisms returned. At first we had no idea why but when we found the empty cake tin we were naturally angry. But we should not have been; he was very remorseful and knew he had been silly. I suppose it was a valuable lesson.

His teachers and tutor are amazed at the transformation. His schoolwork has improved dramatically. He brings home extra work by choice, his concentration span is far longer, and in class he is cheerful and cooperative.

The fraught atmosphere in the home has gone. He is often invited out for tea now and several mothers have approached me and told me what a delight he now is to have in their homes. It's bliss! We still have to shake ourselves to believe that it's true and just how lucky we were to find your clinic. If we hadn't, I'm sure he would have been under the care of a child or educational psychologist, and what would have become of our loved son by now is open to question.

The ironic thing is, before we met you I had always assumed we were having an extremely balanced diet; I think I told you I am a caterer and dietician by profession. I was wrong. All that has changed now. I understand about food allergies and, as a family, our eating habits have changed dramatically. We all look and feel much healthier!

Once again, thank you.

Mrs B

Case no. 4: Eczema

This case concerns Mr Exley, a 41-year-old man with severe eczema, an unpleasant peeling, weeping and cracking condition of the skin. His face was like a mask, and the eczema extended all over his body, worse in some parts than others. He was an architect, and meeting clients caused him intense embarrassment, so much so that he felt like apologising for himself. At its worst the rash was so bad that he had to be wrapped in bandages soaked in cold water to overcome the intense irritation. It had first started about four years before he came to me, and within the first twelve months he had been in trouble: he had then needed to be kept in hospital for three weeks on steroid medication.

These drugs *appear* wonderful at producing a rapid cure, but there is always a sting in the tail: once you start them you can't easily stop them, or the condition will flare up again. You see, they *never* cure, only mask symptoms. That's exactly what happened to Mr Exley. Three weeks after he was sent home, the rash was worse than ever. He did not succeed in abandoning the steroid creams altogether, but managed to cope with his condition, very wretchedly, for over three more years.

Finally, in desperation, he came to see if I could help. In his case there were few corroborating symptoms to suggest the cause of the rash, but I regard eczema as *always* being an ecological-based disease. If anyone needs convincing, take note of the important clue he gave me: each summer when he goes for a long holiday in the sun it clears up completely. (Rest and sunshine is not the reason, as you will read in a later chapter.) This proved that, intrinsically, there was nothing wrong with him or his body – *not a thing*.

All we had to do was locate what substances were causing such unpleasant skin reactions. I thought it highly probable that food was to blame, and I told him so. I explained the plan to him and assured him that though it was tough at first it represented his best road forward. He considered he had nothing to lose by trying and so agreed. He started the diet stage immediately.

This time there was no dramatic improvement on the elimination step. During the withdrawal phase (which you will read about) his skin at times hung off like shreds of tattered wallpaper; but after three weeks, although his skin was somewhat better, I knew we hadn't succeeded fully. Either he was not allergic to the omitted foods or something he was being allowed to continue in his diet did not agree with him. Yet it would have been a terrible mistake to assume he was not reacting to any of the banned foods; in fact, when we tested them several caused a flare-up, namely wheat, egg (very bad), tomato and milk.

We next went on to inquire into several foods we regard as *relatively* safe. (The emphasised word is important because there is no such thing as an absolutely safe food: I have patients who have been made ill by every substance you can name, including such innocent-sounding ones as carrot, lettuce and water.) In Mr Exley's case we came up trumps with pork and lamb. For both of these he followed the outlined test procedure given in this plan, and there was no mistaking the result: it meant several days of feeling unwell with a raw, itchy skin. Avoiding those also, he began to make rapid progress; and within weeks his skin looked clear and healthy except for small patches on his lower legs. Since none of his clients see this part of him it causes no embarrassment or difficulty, and naturally he is very pleased.

Case no. 5: Bowel disorder

The next patient is Maria, an attractive 24-year-old Londoner of Cypriot extraction. She came to see me with abdominal distress, flatulence, bloating and variability of bowel function. Sometimes she would be constipated for days on end; at others she had diarrhoea so severely that she would be caught out and have to run immediately to the nearest toilet. The complaint had troubled her for as long as she could remember; furthermore, her father, *his* father, an aunt and a young cousin were affected in exactly the same way.

Almost continual stomach pains were bad enough, but what troubled her most was the flatulence. She had a job that meant a lot to her: working for a celebrity tour promotion agency. It meant she had frequent opportunities to accompany artistes and stars for up to a day, taking them for meals and showing them around the capital. But so often had she declined these wonderful assignments (using fabricated excuses about 'important appointments') that her employers had assumed she was not interested and ceased to ask her. Instead she was left with mundane office chores, and even then things were sometimes difficult; she had to suddenly excuse herself from a meeting to break wind in the corridor outside.

Her relationships with the opposite sex were spoilt because she was embarrassed about her condition. She had a fixation that she smelt offensive, and one boyfriend, perhaps trying to be helpful, had dropped hints about this, indicating that it was not all 'in her mind'. When the symptoms were particularly bad she preferred to stay at home rather than mix with others, making up feeble excuses. Few men were prepared to put up with her apparent indifference and to persist. Her current boyfriend was a little more understanding, but she refused to see him very often and could not bring herself to tell him why. Naturally, he was puzzled and thought her a strange girl.

Apart from the bowel disorder Maria also occasionally suffered from panic attacks, when everything seemed to press in on her. At these times she would experience the fright of impending doom and feel certain she was about to die. However, her overriding emotion was not anxiety but deep despair and gloom; she frequently felt so depressed that suicide seemed the only answer. Fortunately she had never tried it, otherwise she would have ended up in the hands of some psychiatrist and the outcome might not have been so happy. She had been admitted to hospital twice for investigations, but all tests had proved negative. The final diagnosis (which is no diagnosis at all) was a 'lazy colon', and she was prescribed drugs which failed to help. Disillusioned and cynical, she had long since given up seeing her family doctor.

I inquired into her diet with my routine inventory (see Chapter 4), and she told me she was eating largely wholefoods, including plenty of fruit and vegetables, both fresh and simply cooked. She ate very few tinned and packet meals and no junk food, except on birthdays and at the seaside: on the surface of it, not a very high-risk diet. But then I knew that *any* food was a *potential* allergen.

I explained to Maria that since her digestive tract appeared to bear the brunt of symptoms, food intolerance was very probable. She liked the sound of the approach used in the Food Allergy Plan and decided to give it a try. Within ten days she had made startling progress: the flatulence had ceased completely, her abdominal pains had dropped to a tenth of their former level, and she felt *wonderful*. Her stomach was now flat instead of bloated. Energy and confidence radiated from her. She told me confidentially that her libido was on the increase. The black moods had lifted, and she now considered herself equal to any social or work pressure that might come her way.

From then on she never looked back. Apart from occasions when she deliberately tested a food and experienced a reaction, her symptoms have not returned. Subsequently we found she was allergic to cabbage, cauliflower, turnip (all members of the mustard family), potato, lamb, pork, wheat, egg and tomato. She had been eating one or another of these foods every day yet had never suspected them to be the trouble: none had ever caused an obvious symptom that had aroused her suspicions. Nevertheless, within a few days on this plan, carrying out the correct procedure as outlined by me, she was able to demonstrate a pronounced reaction to each of the above foods. Incidentally, egg seemed to be the cause of most of the flatulence: within minutes of the test dose she was breaking offensive wind – long before any egg could possibly have reached the lower bowel.

Her work is now her greatest pleasure, and she accepts the hostess assignments without hesitation, rubbing shoulders with VIPs and celebrities, at ease and, by all accounts, popular – after all, she knows London better than most native Britons do.

Case no. 6: Schizophrenia

A young man I shall call Tony came to my clinic, and I think it would be no exaggeration to state this his life was in ruins due to unsuspected food allergies. His story has all the human drama you could wish for outside the fantasy annals of Dr Kildare. He came from a good home, had enjoyed normal health as a child, did well at school and at eleven-plus time there had been no clouds on his life's horizon. His secondary education had started off well: he had shown himself to be very bright, and his teachers had expected him to be very successful in the public examinations when he was sixteen.

Then a double tragedy struck: his grandfather, to whom he was very close, died suddenly, and within a very short interval a close friend committed suicide. People die all the time, of course, with varying degrees of impact on those they leave behind; but for an adolescent boy facing the stress of preparation for major examinations it proved rather a lot to cope with. Tony's mood changed, and he began to suffer long bouts of gloom. At times he became so indolent with despondency that it quite worried his parents. They sought medical advice, with the result that at the incredibly early age of fourteen he was put on antidepressant drugs. These are a disaster at any age, in my opinion, but to prescribe them for a newly forming adult personality was an unforgivable blunder.

Despite it all Tony struggled on at school, and few people knew his troubles. There was therefore much consternation and surprise when he failed badly in his O level exams. Doubtless being dosed up on psychotropic (mind-altering) drugs had a lot to do with this. He was allowed to stay on nevertheless, but in the sixth form his behaviour progressively deteriorated: his bouts of depression caused him to become truculent, moody and unreasonable. Finally, even his friends were alienated. At this stage he was diagnosed as a case of schizophrenia.

Sadly, he failed his A level examinations and his promising academic career came to an end. He had been offered a university place on the strength of his known abilities, but was unable to go. Even a most understanding faculty could not permit a student to matriculate without justifiable exam results; it simply would not be fair to other students competing for a place. So Tony ended up working in a library. It was work which held no interest for him and failed to challenge his intellect. There were no prospects that stimulated him, and it was, in every sense, a dead-end job: in other words, in all normal social terms he was a failure, and knew it, which only served to enhance his general mood of depression. Life was a drudge that could only be borne by taking frequent large doses of drugs, and by this time he was having one of these by injection – all this, remember, before he was twenty. What could possibly have gone wrong to snuff out such a promising bright spark?

Actually, there were many clues for the person who knew what to look for: while he was in hospital a skin rash was noticed which passed without comment; he suffered from headaches, palpitations and sudden tiredness after eating; his mood was particularly bad first thing in the morning and breakfast helped him feel better; also, he was occasionally gripped by eating binges. These and other signs made it very obvious to me that Tony had food allergies. He was put on the diet given in Chapter 5 and followed the plan outlined in this book. Within days he began to improve, and within a fortnight an astonishing change had taken place. He described it as being like waking up after years of sleep. His mind cleared as if a fog had lifted, and for the first time in years he was able to look towards the future and feel it was something friendly instead of hostile; for him it was a time of new horizons. He began to reduce the amount of drugs he took. He was a new human being, cheerful and sociable. The nightmare which had begun as a bereavement was finally at an end.

Subsequent tests showed him to be allergic to a wide variety of the foods he had been eating regularly. The worst offenders were cane sugar, milk, cheese, apple, chocolate and tomato, while others included chicken, potato, wheat, egg, yeast and rice – hardly surprising, therefore, that he was ill! Since then he has made plans to restart his studies: there is no question that both his ability to concentrate and the right motivation have returned. Perhaps in a later edition of this book I will be able to report that he finally obtained his degree – who knows?

As I have said, these are just examples of the many, many conditions that can be improved or cured by solving the riddle of food allergies. The list of known diseases that respond is actually a very impressive one. My colleagues and I have a total of hundreds of thousands of cases to prove this. These include patients with mouth ulcers, catarrh, asthma, migraine, epilepsy, diabetes, ulcerative colitis, Crohn's disease, high blood pressure, cystitis (without any evidence of infection), arthritis, eczema, urticaria, peptic ulcer, depression, schizophrenia, anxiety, hyperactivity (in children), mania (in adults), nephrotic syndrome, alcoholism, obesity and menstrual disorders. There are many others besides. In addition there are a large number of complaints which are really no more than symptoms, though there is a tendency to give these fancy names and consider that a 'diagnosis', as in Maria's case above. Examples are irritable bowel syndrome, spastic colon, cardiac arrhythmias, Menière's disease and sexual dysfunction. Finally, there are very many ordinary everyday symptoms, from tiredness and irritability, to forgetfulness and indigestion, which could be caused by allergies. The first table in Chapter 4 lists most of the possibilities.

It is very important to understand that I am not saying that all these conditions are necessarily caused by food and other allergies; simply that they *may* be. It is essential to have a conventional medical check-up in order to exclude the possibility of other, more serious, complaints being the cause of your illness. If they are, get them treated. Only if the diagnosis is vague or the treatment is non-specific or includes drugs and so on as a 'try-out' should you try the approach of this book first.

That's if your condition is a relatively new one. Unfortunately, I am well aware that for many of you infirmity has already meant many years of drugs that don't work, painful operations that were unnecessary, possible ridicule from your doctor and relatives, and finally the ultimate tag that disposes of you as a sufferer by saying that your problems are psychosomatic, that is 'all in the mind'. At least if you have had extensive tests and nothing has been found wrong you can be fairly sure your illness is not organic. That's when allergy testing comes into its own. You are entitled to proceed on this plan without further notice.

How can such simple substances as everyday foods cause so much trouble? Let's advance a chapter and discuss it a little more fully.

2

Orientation and Understanding

This might seem a rather boring title for a chapter; nevertheless, you cannot avoid the need to understand what you are doing if you are to be able to help yourself overcome your allergy problem. There are a great many new discoveries in this field, so even if you have had a great deal of experience of allergies and perhaps feel you know about them, the chances are that you will learn something. What are presented here are really aspects of a new science, clinical ecology, not conventional thinking by established allergists, so do not be discouraged if up to now approaching your illness as an allergy has failed to produce any beneficial result.

DEFINITION TIME

Let's start with a few terms: you can't expect to understand a new topic unless you become familiar with the use of its special words or jargon. To begin with, what do we mean by *allergy*? It is actually not a very straighforward term, though it is used a lot. The word was first coined in 1906 by an Austrian physician, Von Pirquet, so obviously he had the right to say what he meant by it. He specified it as 'An acquired, specific, altered capacity to react to physical substances on the part of the body'.

Note the word *acquired*: it means you do not inherit the sensitivity. According to our understanding of the mechanism, you need to be exposed to the substance before you develop a reaction to it. This exposure may be as slight as one prior contact, yet it must take place. It is confusing, perhaps, that many infants are born with allergies, but that does not violate this stipulation. The fact is that babies in the womb are exposed to a great many potentially allergenic substances via the mother's diet and bloodstream. This is how we think they acquire the sensitivity.

The term *specific* means that the reaction associated with a particular substance is quite unique, even though the results may not be. Thus tomato may make you ill, and so may house dust, but the reacting mechanism in each case is not the same, though the symptom that is caused may well be.

Altered is really a way of saying that it is peculiar to the individual in question, not something that the rest of us are troubled by. This is important, for otherwise we fail to distinguish the special problems of allergy from those of straightforward poisoning. Thus cyanide or muscarine (from the toadstool *Aminita muscaria*) make everyone ill – these are poisons. But some individuals are made ill by simple substances such as milk, coffee and egg, and this is not normal. These foods cause no trouble for the majority of the population, and so, for some people, this is an *altered* (abnormal) reaction.

There is, however, a certain amount of overlap between allergy and poisoning effects: for example, house gas makes us all ill in sufficient concentration, but there are an unlucky few who react even to the tiniest traces of it, traces so small that the concentration will not register on instruments from the gas board. Are they simply being poisoned at an earlier stage, or is this a special *altered* reaction on their part that we may call an allergy? Often it is difficult to decide. But fortunately we do not need to make up our minds between the two phenomena: in the end, if the patient feels better for avoiding that particular substance, *that* is what counts.

Some doctors went on to extend Von Pirquet's work and discovered that *some* allergy reactions were mediated by antibodies (special chemicals provoked by the encounter) and certain lymphocytes, a type of white blood cell – very interesting. Yet this was followed by an insistence that *only* those reactions which involved demonstrable antibodies and/or lymphocytes could be called allergies. This is an extraordinarily narrow and arrogant viewpoint. Other reactions are then dismissed as – what? 'All in the mind' is a common label. It isn't very scientific to dismiss phenomena for which we have no explanation as 'imaginary', and it is especially hurtful to the poor patient, who has not only to bear this insulting jibe but also to continue to suffer the illness because no one will take it seriously.

I have even heard doctors insist that food and chemicals *could not possibly* make people unwell simply because antibodies cannot be shown. They stick to this idiotic viewpoint despite the existence of hundreds of thousands of documented recoveries. Since they believe the patients to be neurotic or 'imagining' their symptoms, their usual explanation for all these astonishing recoveries is that the patient responds because 'someone is taking an interest' in his or her case. (Don't laugh – I have heard this on many occasions.) These gentlemen, and quite a few ladies, are not troubled by mere facts, only by the entrenchment of obscure pet theories.

It often comes as a shock to patients to realise that doctors rarely seem excited and enthusiastic about each new breakthrough in healing. Medicine has a particularly bad history in this respect: almost every new advance has had to be fought for in the teeth of severe opposition. There seems to be a peculiar, almost sinister, aspect to the medical profession that makes it resistant to new ideas. Unfortunately, of course, this works to the detriment of patients, who trustingly believe their own physician to be abreast of new developments without realising that he or she may be actively opposed to an idea *without ever having tried it out personally*.

Well, if you are with me this far you will understand that I don't have much patience with the accepted and 'authoritarian' point of view. Is there an alternative? Fortunately, there is. An increasing number of doctors – and I am very proud to be one – have sloughed off their narrow, formal training. We don't care, when it comes to the crunch, about antibodies, T-cells and 'laboratory reports'; all that counts, to our way of thinking, is 'Does it make the patient ill?'

We extend our critical purview to food, the atmosphere, the water we drink and, yes, even to drugs – so beloved of the medical establishment. In other words, any part of the environment could be potentially harmful to the right sort of person (or the wrong sort, to be logical, I suppose). We call ourselves *clinical ecologists*, and this branch of medical science enjoys the title of *clinical ecology* (ecology: the study of an organism in relation to its environment). We have evolved a practical, *working* definition of an allergy, whether to a food or any other substance. Note that it does not rely on any laboratory test, simply upon *observation of the patient*, sadly a dying art in 'modern' medicine. It is simply this:

A substance is considered to be an allergen if, firstly, the patient feels better on avoiding it; secondly, he or she becomes ill again on re-exposure to it; and thirdly, no other obvious cause for the symptoms can be shown. The first two must be capable of being repeated on more than one occasion. Yet there are certain catches to this which must be understood, or the unwary or casual observer will be tripped up. For example, the patient may not feel better merely by virtue of avoiding one allergy substance. If several others are also causing trouble, why should that person feel well, unless he or she avoids them also?

This is what Dr Doris Rapp, one of the great American ladies of medicine, refers to as the 'eight nails in the shoe' trap. If you have eight nails sticking up in your shoe, you will surely limp. If you draw four or even six of these, it may be no use – you still limp because of the remainder. You need to get rid of all eight for a proper recovery.

Metaphorically speaking, it is the same with allergies. Numerous patients have come to me and explained that they had tried giving up, say, milk for a few weeks and felt no better; therefore they couldn't possibly be allergic to it. To begin with, very few of them succeeded in avoiding milk altogether since it occurs hidden in bread, biscuits, sausages and margarine, for example. The other point is that you have to *avoid enough foods to feel better* before you can infer that you were allergic to any. This will be explained to you in the course of this book and, indeed, is what the Food Allergy Plan is all about! Furthermore, if you do not allow yourself a sufficient amount of time away from the food before testing it you may get no obvious reaction, even from a bad allergy food when you return to it. The explanation for this 'masking' phenomenon is also given later (see Chapter 3). This is probably the biggest single reason why so many people fail to detect their own allergies and why so many doctors are blind to the problem, especially in connection with food.

But allowing for these stumbling blocks, the definition holds good and is very workable: I have used it in my practice for many years now, often with spectacular results. It is a very long time since I prescribed any drugs, except in an emergency; yet I have made more people well and gained more lifelong friends among my patients than in all of my medical career prior to taking up this speciality. It is very satisfying and yet humbling in its simplicity.

HISTORY

The pioneer work in clinical ecology was begun in America in the 1920s. All those who practise it today have cause to be grateful to Dr Albert Rowe Snr., who first experimented with elimination dieting; Dr Herbert Rinkel, who verified the existence of the masked or hidden allergy, which I rate as the biggest medical discovery since anaesthetics and on a par with antibiotics; and who showed us how to rotate and diversify diets (see Chapter 10). Probably the greatest and most revered worker in the field, now the doyen of environmental medicine, is Dr Théron Randolph of Chicago. For years he had to endure the scorn and reprobation of his colleagues: a story of courage and determination full of the very essence of human drama. Yet he persisted and saw his life's work vindicated. His book *Human Ecology and Susceptibility to the Chemical Environment* has become a classic text, and any doctor who has not read it should feel ashamed. Through his continued writings Randolph is probably our greatest voice; yet withal he continues to be an active clinician and researcher, though now almost eighty. Other key names, all American, are Doris Rapp (already mentioned), William Rea, Michael Zeller, William Philpott, William Crook and Marshall Mandell.

Here in Britain Dr Richard Mackarness has flown the flag for us and become a world-renowned name. He began as a consultant psychiatrist at the Park-Prewett Hospital in Basingstoke and, like many of his counterparts from across the Atlantic, took an interest in clinical ecology because he personally was a sufferer. It helped him to a new life, and he realised it could do the same for others. He is now retired, but his influence will continue for many years to come. He is the author of two best-selling books, *Not all in the Mind* and *Chemical Victims* (see Appendix 4). Together with Mrs Amelia Nathan-Hill he founded a British charitable organisation called Action Against Allergy, which aims to promote a wider knowledge of the social and scientific problems connected with allergies (see Appendix 3 for address).

At present there is a great deal of public interest in the subject: every time I speak on the radio or one of our patients hits the headlines we are inundated with inquiries. It is a sad but true fact that the public at large seem to be showing more interest in these exciting new discoveries than the medical profession itself. Yet quite recently signs have emerged that this is changing. Reports of two creditable studies have been published in *The Lancet*, the highly respected medical scientific journal. (Regrettably, most doctors are not in the habit of trying things for themselves and won't believe anything that hasn't been 'proved' by a study that is published in a leading journal.) The first of these (20 November 1982) has become known as 'the Cambridge Study'. Doctors Alun Jones, McLaughlin, Shorthouse, Workman and Hunter, working at Addenbrooks Hospital and the Universtiy of Cambridge showed that foods were able to provoke the symptoms of so-called irritable bowel syndrome in fourteen out of twenty-one patients. This was done double-blind, which means that extraneous factors, due perhaps to the patient knowing what he was being tested with, were ruled out. Irritable bowel syndrome is typical of many 'mysterious' complaints which have kept conventional doctors puzzled for years. In actual fact, clinical ecologists have been saying it was food allergy for decades.

An even more historic step was the publication (October 1983) of the findings of a carefully staged study of migraine in children. Doctors Egger, Carter, Wilson and Turner and Professor Soothil of the Hospital for Sick Children and Institute of Child Care, Great Ormond Street, London, studied eighty-eight youngsters so afflicted. They were able to demonstrate a clear relationship with food and food additives in no fewer than eighty-two of those cases! Quite startling evidence, and very satisfying for clinical ecologists, who have had to bear their colleagues' scorn and indifference while trying to make it known that food and chemical allergies are by far the greatest factor in migraines. It also, of course, helps in the cause of better diets for children and will perhaps lead to eventual legislation against some of the worst offenders among food ingredients – unless manufacturers become more responsible without the need for legal intervention. The important thing about Professor Soothil's study is that it showed a clear understanding of the principles of clinical ecology as outlined in this book. Far too often studies have ignored the true mechanics of *how* an allergic substance behaves in the body, failed to get results, and then said 'No such thing as allergies' when all that has really been proved is that the investigator doesn't have a clue about what he or she is up against.

This was the trouble with an otherwise worthy attempt to study the possible link between food allergies and mental illness carried out by Doctors Pearson, Rix and Bentley at Withington Hospital, Manchester. The patients were put on a fast but not taken to the point at which their symptoms cleared. The possibility of concomitant chemical allergies was not considered, which means that in some patients the symptoms may never have cleared simply on a fast. Thus all further tests were meaningless because the patient still had his or her symptoms (see Chapter 8 for more information on the correct way to carry out fast tests). Also, the challenges involved were carried out by feeding patients foodstuffs in capsule form, a situation which clearly bears no relationship to what happens when a patient actually *eats* the food. The conclusion of this poorly worked out study was that most of the twenty-three patients studied had symptoms which were 'all in the mind', a depressing and common conclusion which helps no one, belittles the patient and is most often simply quite wrong. If the study actually proved anything, it was one of two points: either that some patients may not respond to food allergies but that their problems *could* be chemical allergies, or that the investigators didn't understand what they were up against.

While the controversy rages, your own GP could be forgiven for not making up his or her mind definitely, but not for being totally and blindly opposed to the possibility of ecology disease (which far too many of them are), or for ignoring the numerous successful cures and failing to at least try the methods given here when he or she has little or nothing else to offer. This is in fact a very safe and simple approach, far more so than modern drugs, and it does no one any harm to try it. The reality is, however, that for many years to come food allergy sufferers may be unable to get the kind of help they need from their own doctors. Experience shows that this is a very common condition, and not rare as was once thought. Thus there will be many people who simply do not know where to turn for help.

Fortunately, it is a subject that lends itself well to the have-a-go-yourself approach. Given a minimum of information, such as that supplied here by me, any individual of average intelligence ought to be able to sort himself or herself out if food allergies are the cause of the trouble. There is a lengthy self-evaluation section which should enable you to find out whether or not this applies to you. If it does, good luck with the book: you may be a new person by the time you reach the last chapter!

It has been estimated that the National Health Service, yearly teetering on the verge of bankruptcy, could save itself thousands of millions of pounds annually by paying attention to what clinical ecologists are telling them and applying it. Probably 50 per cent of all patients who attend a doctor have a condition which is partly or wholly caused by food and other allergies. The very sufferers who go back time and time again, trying everyone's patience and running up huge bills for treatment and drugs but never becoming truly well, are the ones most likely to be victims of this phenomenon. Yet, given the right approach, they needn't be ill at all.

Often an expensive series of tests and investigations leads nowhere. The disease remains as baffling and elusive as it was in the first place. This leads to newer and stranger 'diagnoses' that are not really diagnoses at all, such as the so-called irritable bowel syndrome. The waste of money is staggering. Do we go further in this direction − or has the time come to review our strategy and change paths? It would surely be much more sensible to start patients off with a change of diet, and then, only if *that* doesn't help, to engage in these costly and time-consuming procedures.

If this book helps even one of the sufferers, I shall be very pleased. I make no claim to original discoveries in clinical ecology, but the method given here is my own, developed over a number of years. I use it daily, so I know it works. My practice goes far beyond this plan, but it still forms a very important fundamental part of it.

FOOD ALLERGIES

There are many aspects to clinical ecology, yet this little book is concerned almost entirely with food allergies. Why are these so important? Simply because they are so common: other substances have their effects, but food assumes a leading place in the table of troublemakers because we are intimate with such large quantities of it. Think of the volume of food you put *inside* your body each day, and compare that with the tiny traces of pollen in the air in springtime. Nevertheless, as hay fever victims know, it takes only small amounts of pollen to make someone very ill indeed. In fact, food reactions seem to have been increasing in recent years. This is almost certainly a reflection on our deteriorating diets, which contain larger quantities of carbohydrate and chemicals than formerly. Yet these are precisely the sort of foods which cause most allergy reactions!

Just how common are allergies? Did our ancestors have them? These are questions I am often asked. The answer to the first can be simply put: there are many individuals who have a few allergies and a few individuals who have many allergies. It is the latter group who tend to become ill, and most of my patients belong to it. But if you cared to stop people in the street at random and questioned them closely enough, most of them would be able to report at least one food that disagreed with them in some way, whether so slightly as to cause no more than flatulence or badly enough to cause vomiting. If the problem is a very minor one and general health is good, few people give such reactions a second thought; they are considered almost 'normal'. The answer to the second question will take a little longer.

WHAT DID CAVEMEN EAT?

To understand this more fully it is necessary to inquire into what we *should* eat. Dr Richard Mackarness, in *Not all in the Mind* (see Appendix 4) calls our attention to the archaeological view of diet. A little study in this direction suggests that primitive man's natural foods were fruit, vegetables and – when he could get them – meat or fish. There was no cereal products such as bread (from wheat); dairy produce was unknown beyond infancy; and stimulant drinks (such as tea and coffee), sugar and other modern foods did not form part of this diet. It is only a supposition, but I think a reasonable one, that their daily foods would have suited early *Homo sapiens* and his immediate progeny: presumably nature, through the process of natural selection, would have got the balance about right.

Yet today we consume predominantly cereal foods (bread, cakes, biscuits, pastry, and so on), dairy produce (milk, butter, cream, cheese and yoghurt), sugar, eggs and stimulant drinks. If the Stone Age diet theory is correct, all these are most unnatural. It would therefore not be surprising if eating as we do tended to cause ill health. Adverse reactions to foods, in other words food allergies, would occur in direct proportion to the level of deterioration in our food, and that seems to be precisely what has happened: the less 'biological' food we eat, such as meat, fruit and vegetables, the more illness we are prone to as a direct consequence of our diet.

Currently there is a great deal of public interest in the high fibre diet. We may even be in the grip of 'fibre fever', as Dr Stephen Davies has described it. I personally believe that fibre is a red herring and that the real success of such a diet comes from the necessary reversal to more natural and whole foods higher in the vitamins and minerals which are usually removed by processing. Interestingly, quite a few people are made ill by the high fibre diet, and for all the cases I have reviewed that turned out be due to wheat intolerance. With its emphasis on wholemeal bread and bran (a wheat derivative) the high fibre diet is very tough on wheat-allergic patients, and it so happens that it is probably the commonest of all food allergies. Though there are certain helpful nutrients in wheatgerm, it can hardly be a safe food for those who are made ill by it. The fact that it is capable of producing adverse effects tends to support the 'caveman' view of healthy eating.

Milk is another diet impostor. To listen to all the propaganda you would get the impression that anyone who didn't drink at least a pint of it a day was inevitably doomed to ill health. In fact, the opposite is probably true: millions of humans drink no milk at all and experience no deficiencies as a result, but a great many are made sick, without knowing it, by a milk allergy. Children suffer particularly in this respect. Pumped full of milk to 'do them good', many are victims of severe milk allergy and so are constantly poorly with sore throats, runny noses, earache, 'teething troubles', colic and a whole host of other childhood complaints which magically disappear when that substance is removed from their diet. The fact is that milk is not a natural food: no animal in nature drinks milk after its infancy, and it is completely illogical to suppose that man must be different.

If you pause to think for a moment you will realise that grains, dairy food and other farm produce such as eggs have only been in our diet since we settled the land and became civilised. Whereas there are many who would argue that civilisation has not yet arrived, scholars would date this only from about ten thousand years ago – far more recently than you would think. In biology, where evolutionary changes take place slowly over millions of years, such a short time span is a drop in the ocean. In other words, we simply haven't had time to *adapt* to these new foodstuffs, and as a result don't handle them well on ingestion. They are still alien foods so far as the cells of our body are concerned: our palate may be in the twentieth century, but our constitution is still that of a forest-dwelling higher ape. (This may be shocking to dedicated gourmets!)

THE ADULTERATION OF FOOD

But we have been eating cereals and milk for centuries, you say. True. And probably this has enabled most of us to tolerate such foods, all other things being equal. But other factors have now been brought into the fray. Look at what has been happening to food in the last fifty years, especially the last twenty-five: now we have *chemical* food additives. Most of these have come into use on the present vast scale only since the last war, yet in just a few decades this adulteration of our basic foods has reached absurd proportions. Take a walk round any super-market and look at the products on the shelves: it is almost impossible to buy simple, plain food. There are added colourants, emulsifiers, preservatives, flavour enhancers and scores of other alien ingredients that *no one* has had time to adapt to.

There are over 3,000 such substances available and over 1,100 are listed for legal use in the United Kingdom. Individually, these are supposed to be harmless up to the permitted levels; but in reality this is nonsense. It fails to take into account two very important points: firstly, normal human variation, mentioned earlier, which means that what may be quite safe for the majority of us can make some unlucky, sensitive people very ill indeed; secondly, the fact that chemical additives are never used singly. When several occur together in the same mixture, who is to say that the many and complex relationships between each of the separate items do not result in a harmful or even poisonous combination? I have talked to food chemists on this point and received no satisfactory answer.

Then there are toxic substances, such as insecticides and fertilisers, that are sprayed onto crops before harvesting and eating. There is a vast array of chemicals in the armoury of the modern farmer or market gardener, almost all of which are as inimical to human life as they are to six-legged forms. The medical effects of these substances have not been fully studied, even in relation to acute poisoning episodes, never mind chronic exposure. The chemical manufacturing companies have, of course, no incentive to do so, and government departments, like sailors setting to sea without maps and compass, are blind to the danger and will not see until it is tragically too late – too late for some and not soon enough for the many. Instead, like profligate fools, we squander our precious environment, poisoning and polluting it until we ourselves, and more especially our children, are doomed to suffer the consequences unless something is done to halt the madness.

One of my patients is a farmer's wife, and she tells me that she and her family wouldn't *dream* of eating the food they send to market for others to consume. 'It's poisoned!' she declares, and she should know since she and her husband are only too well aware of the abuses concerned. Instead, they grow their own food in a special plot without using chemicals. Like many farmers, they feel a keen economic pressure to use artificial methods to increase their yield. The irony of this is that 'organic' farming methods have been researched and advanced to the point where there is no advantage in using chemicals. Unfortunately, this is not widely known: big business controls most of the communications and media, and doubtless slick selling and commercialism will see to it that all but the most studious of farmers never hear about these advances in natural methods but will instead be told, in glowing terms, of all that the wonders of science can do for them financially (See Henry Doubleday Research Organization, Appendices 2 and 3). I worked briefly as company doctor to a major British food manufacturer involved in the making of convenience meats. One of the chemicals added to the sausage mixture was so noxious that if any of the operatives accidentally came into contact with the powder he or she would end up at the first-aid station with burning skin and painful weeping eyes; yet this substance is a legally permitted food additive.

Wheat-cropping is now big business for some British farmers. Because high prices are guaranteed by the EEC – even though we have far more wheat than we consume – it pays to invest heavily in yield. It is commercially viable to spray the crop eight or ten times before harvesting, so absurdly high are the sales returns. This may include treatments with weedkillers, fungicides, fertilisers and insecticides. The irony of it that is we in Europe have metaphorical 'wheat mountains': vast stores of unconsumed grain that nobody wants.

Of course, all these chemicals are present on the wheat at the moment of harvesting; indeed, there is no way of removing it. So whole-wheat, beloved of the health food fan, is a far from wholesome product to eat on this account. I could go on at length, but I'm sure you understand the overall idea: that our diets are now *loaded* with a great many unnatural substances that nature never intended us to eat. This in turn reduces our ability to deal with other, not-so-natural foodstuffs such as grains and dairy produce. Our bodies are having demands laid on them which for many of us cannot be met.

Man is very adaptable; you only have to look at his staggering conquests of nature to realise that. Yet it takes time to accommodate a new food into our diets. Given a few hundred thousands years, we might easily be able to consume burgers and cola without any ill effects – I only we hope that we as a species do not have the folly to persist with such fare!

THE FIRST CASUALTIES

Many people are ill today who could reasonably have expected not to be fifty years ago. They are not unwell in the strict sense as there is nothing wrong with them; it is just that the environment is too hostile and they are being slowly poisoned by it, thus they experience symptoms and all the apparent signs of disease. Medical science has hitherto been unable to help them, simply because within its parameters many of them are seen as having nothing demonstrably wrong with them.

I don't think I'm going out on a limb when I say that as a species (more exactly as the subspecies of *Homo sapiens* that is 'Westernised') we are far less healthy than we used to be. It is depressingly rare to find people who are 100 per cent fit, and almost unheard of outside the young adult group. In this sense, none of us are coping very well with the egregious demands of our technicalised environment. It seems to be simply that some are falling victim to it sooner and more completely than others; not that this vulnerable group are in essence different from the rest.

Wholefood eating is, rightly, becoming popular. Those who practise it feel better, largely because such a diet drastically reduces the amount of chemical exposure through eating. It leaves the problems of atmospheric and water pollution unresolved, but is a major step in the right direction. Food has a large part to play simply because of the relatively great amounts of it we consume. A word of warning, however, before you rush out to the health food shop: read the rest of this book first, otherwise it is possible to make serious mistakes. Health foods may make you ill because of your allergies; first you need to know which foods suit you and which do not. This book is actually a unique dietary approach in that it shows you how to work out a completely personal diet, one which is right for you and you alone. No matter how nutritious a food is you will not recover while eating it if you are allergic to it. This gives rise to some strange anomalies. People sometimes look at me as if I am slightly mad when I say white bread can be better for you than brown, but the fact is that for wheat-allergic patients this is true. Good nutrition may have other pitfalls. Finish reading first, and then see what you think.

A FRIGHTENING EXPERIMENT

Between 1932 and 1942 Dr Francis M. Pottenger conducted a number of nutritional experiments on cats. Certain animals were put on diets consisting only of treated and cooked foods equivalent to our processed foods and quite unlike the normal, healthy cat diet of raw meat. Predictably, they became ill, and by the third generation were so effete as to be infertile so that those particular strains died out. But what was really disturbing was the fact that cats taken off the deficient diet *took three generations to return to normal health parameters*. Parallels with our modern human diets are inevitable, and if the findings hold true for us as well as for cats the implications are very serious indeed: namely that through bad eating we are ruining not only our own health but also that of our children and grandchildren.

Unfortunately, this very important study has gone largely ignored by the medical establishment. There are several reasons for this: to begin with, the medical profession as a whole tends to ignore nutrition as being relevant to health; secondly, although this experiment was a milestone and undoubtedly years ahead of its time, it failed to conform to current criteria in medical scientific rhetoric. I may also be forgiven a certain amount of cynicism in saying that since the findings were counter to the interests of big business Pottenger's work was doomed to hostility.

Pottenger's oblique condemnation of our modern human fare

is similar to the conclusions drawn by Sir Robert McCarrison from his studies of nutrition in rats. The work of these two men has been backed up by many later experiments and results; but once again the medical fraternity, hidebound by its adherence to restrictive scientific precepts, ignores the findings as 'unproven'. Considering the enormous implications to our health and longevity, one can only describe this ostrich-like attitude as foolish in the extreme. Even if the criticism of the original method were justified, one would expect to see some of the enormous amount of money currently devoted to developing newer and yet more powerful (harmful) drugs being spent on repeating the tests in a manner that would satisfy the most fastidious critic.

Interestingly, the work of both scientists has been kept alive by an enclave of convinced supporters in the form of the McCarrison Society of Great Britain and the Price-Pottenger Nutrition Foundation in the USA. For the addresses and details of these two worthy organisations, see Appendix 3.

ARE ALLERGIES HEREDITARY?

This is a question that is often asked, and the answer must be guarded until more exact knowledge becomes available. Certainly the problems do run in families, but that does not point to a gene inheritance *per se*. Think of the cats experiment just quoted above. If parents tend to eat poorly and make themselves ill due to maladaptation to foods, the chances are they will do the same to their offspring. The youngsters will tend to pick up the same cooking and eating pattern and pass it on to *their* children, and so the trend continues. Thus allergies may *appear* to be inherited without actually being so. The picture is further complicated by the fact that a great many babies are now being born with frank allergies. In many cases this is due to exposure to allergenic foods *in utero*. Here the child certainly has congenital allergies, but once again did not 'inherit' them in the exact meaning of the word.

I believe the tendency *is* inherited. Statistics suggest that if one parent is affected by allergies the child has a somewhat higher than 50 per cent chance of being affected also. If both parents are cases, that likelihood rises to about 85 per cent –

approaching certainty. Exactly *what* those allergies are, however, depends largely on what you come into contact with, *not*
on what your parents reacted to; thus if a mother has a milk
allergy and avoids milk while pregnant, this is unlikely to
become her child's allergy. Similarly, the resultant illness may
be different: one parent may have asthma, the other eczema,
and yet the child has, say, colitis. You will read later about
'target organs' and why there is so much variation from one
person to the next, even with the same condition, or – more
baffling until you understand the reasons for it – even from day
to day in the *same person*.

DOES THIS MEAN THERE IS NO HOPE?

Of course not: hundreds of thousands of cases prove that a
person can become well again by eliminating allergy foods,
even if he or she was born with a strong allergic sensitivity. In
this book you will be shown first of all how to establish
whether or not you might be suffering from allergies to food
and other substances. It also explains what you can do about it
if you are and how to proceed. The results are well worth
while, and in many cases it means the end of decades or even a
lifetime of suffering. To the rejoicing patient it can indeed seem
like a miracle.

It is sometimes possible to speak of a cure, but we must be
careful with our words. Illnesses such as diabetes, arthritis and
migraine do indeed disappear, never to return, and drugs are no
longer required. In that sense we are speaking of a cure. But the
allergy tendency does not disappear; if you were born with it
you are stuck with it, though fortunately it is possible to
mitigate its worst aspects through the intelligent use of vitamin
and mineral supplements, good food and the avoidance of
obvious triggering factors. You can help the body in its fight,
but the truth is that if you are such an individual you may
always need to be careful about what you eat and drink; some
offending foods may be better left alone altogether. Yet such a
price is a small one to pay for the return of your health, zest
and well-being.

Don't let the example of the cats experiment frighten you
into thinking that damage, once done, is irreversible. It

underlines a problem which we certainly have to face but does not pose a complete barrier to the taking of proper action. That the damage has been done may be a fact, but nature has given us wonderful powers of recovery, and it is amazing how complete the return to normality can be, even in extreme cases.

We must think also of the younger generation and those generations yet to come. We cannot abandon our responsibility to them. If that means changing from our present indulgent habits, ceasing to put cravings and intoxication before health, and building back our own health even if it requires effort that we are no longer used to, then so be it. Health is a precious commodity, especially when you have already lost it, and should not be frittered away. Ignorance may be an excuse, but with the publication of this and similar books on ecology there is really no longer any reason for ignorance; only sloth can maintain your inaction.

Well, that sounded rather like a sermon, didn't it? But, really, the unravelling of the plot can be a lot of fun. Check through the summary to make sure you haven't missed any points, and then let's turn to the next chapter and get down to brass tacks.

SUMMARY

- **An allergy** is an abnormal reaction on the part of the body to some foreign substance, which can be a food. Each reaction is unique, but the resulting symptoms can be similar.
- **Clinical ecologist:** A doctor who makes a special study of the way in which environmental factors – that is, reasons existing *outside* your body – can make you ill.
- **Ecology:** The study of an organism in relation to its environment.
- The meaning of the word 'allergy' is contentious but to a clinical ecologist a substance is an allergen if (1) you feel better by avoiding it; (2) it makes you ill when you re-expose yourself to it; and (3) no other cause can be shown. (Mental symptoms are excluded as a 'cause' as they are usually just another manifestation of the allergy.)
- Food allergies are far commoner than was once supposed.

● We believe that man's natural diet probably consisted of meat, fish, fruit and vegetables. All other foods are relatively new, and as a species we are not yet adapted to them.

3

The Hidden Allergy

The hidden or masked allergy has aptly been called 'the unsuspected enemy' (see Appendix 4). This great contribution to medical science was made by Herbert Rinkel, an American doctor of great acumen and ability who discovered himself to be allergic to eggs despite eating large quantities of them. (His father was a farmer and kept him well supplied for years as an indigent student.) He had avoided them for several days as a test and felt better, but the clinch came when he next ate one and passed out! He was able to reason out the mechanism involved: yet another case of a chance observation grasped upon by a brilliant mind which comprehends significances that most ordinary people would pass by. An understanding of exactly how a hidden allergy works is of vital importance to you in solving your own case. The explanation that follows is given in terms of food allergy, but it is important to remember that the same principles apply to chemical and other sensitivities as well.

Everyone has heard of unfortunate people who come out in a rash after eating strawberries or shellfish. That's a food allergy, of course. But really it is no problem: they know they should keep off strawberries or whatever the offending food is, and that is usually the end of it. The real breakthrough came with the realisation that you can be made ill by a food *without knowing it is doing it*. Hence the name 'hidden' allergy. This has opened the door to cure in countless cases where formerly the real culprit was never even dreamt of.

Suppose you are allergic to egg (it happens to be a very common allergy) and ate it almost every day: bacon and eggs for breakfast each morning, perhaps. For long periods you

39

might feel quite well; then you have a sudden attack of your complaint. You would say to yourself, not unreasonably: 'It can't be egg. I ate it last week *and* the week before and I didn't have any symptoms!' But if this was a *hidden* allergy you would be quite wrong: that's exactly how it could behave. Perhaps you might become suspicious of egg and decide to have a three-egg omelette just to see if you can prove you are sensitive to it. Nothing happens. You might even have your best day for weeks. It's all very baffling, and not surprisingly it was a long while before this mechanism was fully understood, even now it defeats the careless or casual observer. It simply doesn't work to 'eat something and see'.

Is it possible to uncover hidden allergies, except by mere chance? Luckily, it is. That is what this entire book is about, and by the time you have finished it I hope you will be adept at overcoming the barriers to detection at least most of the time, if not always. To start with, there are two very useful clues which point the way to what we are looking for. In order for an allergy to hide or mask, the victim must eat the food with a certain minimum frequency. By experience I find this to be about twice a week, though the exact interval varies from person to person. If you ate the culprit food only occasionally, you would have your attack only once in a while and the chances are it wouldn't take you long to work out what was happening. This is precisely the reason allergies to strawberries and shrimps are so notorious: most of us eat these foods only a few times a year. The body doesn't get the chance to develop a hidden allergy, so there is never any doubt about the severity of the reaction. The real troublemakers are foods eaten frequently, often daily. It is as if the body learns to cope with the problem, and we sometimes speak of becoming 'adapted' to an allergen. 'Maladapted' is the opposite and denotes the periods when it makes you unavoidably ill.

The reason twice a week is an important interval in maintaining a hidden allergy from view has to do with bowel habit. It takes about four days to empty the 'average' bowel (silly term, that), and if a food is eaten more frequently this means it is permanently within the body. People vary, of course. For someone with chronic diarrhoea, the interval may be shorter; constipation, on the other hand, increases it. What matters is that the masking effect relies on the previous dose being already there at the point when a food is eaten. This is logical: if there is milk already present and the symptoms are in abeyance, drinking milk shouldn't provoke any. This protection only seems to fail in very advanced cases where the allergy is severe and chronic.

The second *big* clue is that patients tend to get hooked on their allergens (allergen: a substance which causes an allergy reaction). This is an aspect of the problem that intrigues patients and public alike. I'm talking now about real addiction: if the patient goes too long without that food or substance, symptoms begin which induce a craving. More of the food puts an end to the symptoms temporarily, and the craving ceases for a time. Thus the food or drink appears to give a 'lift', but you must understand that this is only because it is causing a 'down' in the first place. You may know someone who always feels better for a cup of tea or a biscuit; it is possible to see such people visibly perk up. That's addiction at work, and, I need hardly point out, it is very common! The mechanism is in no way different from the addiction of a junkie to heroin, or of an alcoholic to liquor. Neither, in certain cases, are the consequences any less drastic — it's just a socially more acceptable addiction, that's all.

Patients sometimes say to me at the clinic, 'Doctor, I'll give up anything you say — as long as it isn't bread!' (for bread read tea, sugar, milk, coffee, potatoes, and so on). Immediately, of course, I suspect that this is something they are going to *have* to give up in order to get well. Sometimes I am accused of being puritanical by my patients: to them it seems I am bent on stopping the things they enjoy and crave the most, and often they are right. Usually this is no more than a jocular criticism, but there are occasions when I am faced with raw, steamy emotion. I have to explain that it is not my fault the situation has come about; I merely have to treat the after-effect of years, even a lifetime, of wrong eating habits.

It is interesting to note in passing that patients at the migraine clinic in London are told not to go more than a few hours without food. To do so often provokes an attack of migraine and you, dear reader, now know why! But I find it baffling and frustrating that the doctors concerned, who are aware of its withdrawal effect, never make the mental leap to recognising they are dealing with an addiction. The very thing that causes a headache on withdrawal is something the patient should avoid completely. There will be one bad headache, but it will clear eventually in the same way that an alcoholic sooner or later gets over the DTs; after that a headache due to that particular cause will not return as long as the food is avoided. (Alcoholics, by the way, *all* have hidden allergies. Whatever the underlying psychosis, and there usually is one, food allergy is the mechanism: see Chapters 12 and 13.)

This addiction mechanism gives rise to another important new term, the *masked allergy*. Essentially, this is the same as a hidden allergy, but it reminds us that in this instance the allergen helps to keep the symptom at bay: in other words, it masks the withdrawal effect, provided it is taken often enough. How often is enough? The interval can vary from as little as one or two hours to forty-eight hours or more; on rare occasions it can exceed seventy-two hours. Remember that if you suffer from constipation or diarrhoea these intervals can vary up or down. I have seen patients who start getting a headache and feeling depressed if they don't get a cup of coffee every hour on the hour, but that is exceptional – I'm sure it doesn't apply to you!

To conclude this chapter let's indulge in a little thoery. Since you are going to have to rescue yourself using the information in this book it is important that you get as full a grasp as possible on the subject. Now, theories are all very well as long as you don't confuse them with facts; they are unproven notions, that is all. We understand very little about how allergies are caused, but that doesn't mean we can't be of practical help. Vaccination was in use for over 200 years before the virus was discovered and the mechanism of immunity understood.

ENZYMES

Personally, I think intolerances are due to damaged or incomplete enzyme systems within the body. Our chemistry is extremely complex, and yet, in health, a balanced, integral whole. Each one of the millions of individual reactions that take place within the body cells requires an enzyme, that is a speeding-up factor. These unusual chemicals are very important to us. Many are known and the reactions they assist with well understood, but there must be countless others waiting to be discovered of whose actions we at present know nothing.

Lack of an enzyme can cause disease. For example, a deficiency of lactose, an enzyme which digests milk, is a well-known cause of illness which is in effect a food allergy or intolerance (though it won't mask). An enzyme called glucose-6-dehydrogenase is lacking in certain individuals and is associated with a certain rare anaemia.

One thing we do know about enzymes is that they poison easily: too much, even trace amounts, of the wrong thing can stop them working. Cyanide poisoning actually works by incapacitating our respiratory or oxygen-using enzymes; *very* tiny quantities do it, which is why cyanide is such a lethal poison. When you think of all the chemicals we breathe, eat and drink it would be surprising if we were *not* damaging our enzymes and impairing their ability to perform correctly and efficiently. It is impossible to predict what the effects will be in a given situation; all we can be sure of is that the results will be far-reaching and harmful. Interference with enzyme systems will lead to, among many things, a greater intolerance of *other* chemicals. Foods are basically chemicals and are digested by enzymes – different ones for fat, starches, sugar, protein and so on – so it is to be expected, really, that an inability to deal properly with foods is a consequence of the widespread presence in the environment of toxic substances.

VITAMINS AND MINERALS

Most enzymes are, moreover, derived from vitamins. A lack of these vital trace substances thus leads to enzyme deficiency and imbalance. This at least is understood to some extent; what is less fully worked out, however, is the role of certain minerals such as zinc, manganese and selenium. Proof is forthcoming that deficiencies of such elements can cause overt and cryptic disease. For example, cobalt, contained in vitamin B12, is necessary for the formation of the red blood pigment that carries oxygen in the blood; a lack of it leads to anaemia. Zinc appears to be important for tissue growth and healing, carbohydrate metabolism, a healthy heart and muscle, protein synthesis and the reduction of atherosclerosis. A proper balance of zinc to copper seems to play a vital role in protection against allergies.

More is being learned about trace elements (as they are called) all the time. When I studied nutrition at medical school these substances were tossed off in a page of the textbook; nowadays there is enough known to fill a sizeable volume. There can be no doubt, even at this stage of budding knowledge, that many of these minerals are *essential* to a proper functioning of body chemistry. Yet our diets are woefully inadequate in many vitamins and minerals; even 'wholefoods' may not provide sufficient of them. Zinc, for example, is deficient even in the soil of Western Europe, never mind in the produce grown on it. Farmers don't supplement it in the earth because a lack of it doesn't affect the yield. Wheat and corn, the commonest ingredients of 'junk' food, contain substances known as phytates which inhibit zinc, so poor eating will further reduce the available amount of this valuable element. Not surprisingly, therefore, zinc deficiency has become a diagnosable entity for those practitioners who know what to look for.

Well, all this in connection with allergies is speculation: you can please yourself whether you believe it or not until the proofs are tied up tightly. It isn't a bad explanation, though, because it is both plausible and fits the facts. If I am correct, then you would predict that illness will get worse as our diets deteriorate and we are exposed to more and more chemicals through food, water and the atmosphere – which, if you've been paying attention, is precisely what I have pointed out *is* happening!

THE THEORY OF ADAPTATION

A different theory – almost a philosophy – which doesn't clash with any of the above is offered by Hans Selye in his General Adaptation Syndrome. If you haven't read his very able book *The Stress of Life* (see Appendix 4), you should. He postulates three stages in coping with stress. This progression would be exhibited by any organism in response to any form of stress, from an amoeba living in slightly tainted water all the way to a pressurized executive in a demanding, harrassing job that is giving him ulcers.

At first the organism reacts strongly to the new stimulus: it fights it, and it is this struggle that the body recognises as symptoms. In human terms, the organism would feel ill. Hippocrates called it the *ponos*, or strife, of disease, and without it no disease exists. Gradually, adaptation occurs. The organism learns to cope with the problem. The symptoms reduce or disappear, and the disease submerges; the human subject feels well again. Selye recognises this as a separate aspect: Stage 2. Yet all the while an insidious attack is taking place. This steadily erodes the body's defences until eventually they are exhausted. The process may take months or decades, but it advances inexorably as long as the stress is present. Finally, when the body can simply cope no more, symptoms re-emerge, and this is Stage 3. The organism is sick, as before, but now in difficulties because there are no defences left. This is the stage of chronic illness.

It is an attractive theory and fits many observations I have made among sick people. It also parallels very closely the histories of allergy sufferers, which is why it is of special interest to us. Many people I question can remember being made ill by certain foods as children: their parents insisted they ate them because 'They are good for you'. In time they were tolerated (the person became adapted to them: Stage 2); but now, years later, the unlucky individual is sick with asthma, arthritis, migraine or any one of a host of diseases and often we track down these very foods as being the cause of the problem. This is Stage 3, and the body has no resistance left so the condition is chronic. Incidentally, the mechanism of addiction to a food coincides with Stage 3: not only is the patient unable to oppose the food physically, but it is as if he or she is unable to oppose it mentally either and has to have it.

Many allergy-based illnesses come on or get worse after periods of acute stress such as an episode of a severe infective disease, bereavement, divorce or redundancy. This is good supportive evidence of the general adaptation theory. It is as if the extra burden becomes too great for the body, already under chemical siege, which then moves rapidly into Stage 3. It could cope – barely – but not in the face of extra stress. Unfortunately, patients often do not recover once the stress is removed again; after the allergies have been triggered, so to speak, they cause illness in their own right. This disease is further stress, which causes further illness, and a vicious circle seems to come about with the result that the patient may still be ill *years* after, say, his or her father died, even though that was what seemed to have brought it on in the first place. This is important because it is a situation from which the only escape seems to be solving the allergies.

The final supportive evidence for Selye's theory – remember it is only a theory, not a proven fact – is the following observation: *the more you eat of a food the more likely you are to develop a maladaptation to it.* Overeating a substance will cause it to disagree with you. The food itself becomes a stress and will accelerate Stage 3.

This is almost certainly the reason why wheat, milk and sugar and so on are such common allergies. Not only are they not really 'natural' foods, which makes them stressful, but they are considerably overconsumed by the population as a whole. Most diets are heavily loaded with bread, milk, sweeteners and cereal products. This may suit the fast-food chains, but I doubt if Mother Nature is amused.

STRESS

Selye's theory extends well beyond food allergies in its scope. Stress is everywhere. If you are under considerable pressure at work, your long-term health is at risk. You should stop to consider the implications of this. In our present society, high in unemployment, you may not feel it is practical to change your job. Nevertheless, you cannot afford to ignore the hazards. If you are under that sort of stress, it is important not to aggravate it in other ways; thus a proper, low-allergy diet could be of vital concern to you. If there are additional factors, such as marital difficulties or financial worries, it is important that you follow closely the rules of good eating given in this book. To work all hours, rest poorly, omit vitamin supplements and then load your system with potentially toxic foods is a certain road to ulcers and heart attacks. I know that for sure, and, believe me, many patients have walked down that road before you, never to return.

SUMMARY

Before we go on, let's have a quick check using a summary of the definitions you have encountered. It will help to make sure you understand the concepts involved:

- **Allergen:** A substance which provokes an allergy reaction.
- **Hidden allergy:** An allergy that doesn't make itself obvious. Constant exposure to it blurs the cause-and-effect relationship.
- **Masked allergy:** The definition of hidden allergy applies, but with the addition of the withdrawal effect. If the person goes too long without that food or substance, symptoms begin which are relieved by the next dose.
- **Addiction:** The need to continue taking a substance because physical discomfort results from being without it.
- **Adaptation:** The body can cope with this substance without experiencing symptoms.
- **Maladaptation:** The body can no longer cope with this substance, and symptoms result.

Right, if you are well braced with a dose of theory telling you why all this is important, read on and let's see what we can do about it.

4

Self-Inventory

First of all, let's find out where you are starting from: what is your present state of health, really? A lot of people are inclined to minimise symptoms and shrug them off. Perhaps this is due to a fear of admitting something is wrong; or simply to the fact that the body adapts so wonderfully, compensating for defects, that the illness steals up on it unnoticed. The latter would explain why some patients only report to the doctor when they are critically ill and disease has progressed much too far. It is important to realise that by the time symptoms do begin it means that this very extensive ability to compensate has already become exhausted. Nature cannot cope any longer, so the matter has become serious. A symptom, no matter how slight, is the body's way of crying out 'Help!'

YOUR CASE HISTORY

Think of this chapter as a case-book on yourself. We are going to open a dossier and fill it with as much relevant information as we can gather through the pages of this book. It will be something to refer to later – to alter and extend, perhaps. That way you may judge your progress or lack of it. Much of what follows is simply good detective work. Well, unlike the inspirational genius of Sherlock Holmes, most crime-solving is really done by the accumulation of sufficient valid data: it takes method and good records.

GENERAL QUESTIONS

Start by answering these generalised questions. From the notes attached to each question you may be able to deduce that you have a strong tendency to suffer from allergies or ecological illness:

1 Do you suffer, or have you ever suffered, from *known* allergies? This can include reactions to food, fumes, pollens, animal danders, dust, moulds, chemicals, metals – in fact, to anything at all. If the answer is 'Yes', then you are certainly in line for more of this kind of trouble.

2 Does anyone in your immediate family (parents, brothers, sisters, aunts, uncles, grandparents, and so on) suffer from any known allergies to anything? If the answer is 'Yes', then again you are at risk of allergy trouble yourself. If you recall the last chapter, we think the *tendency* is inherited. The chances of being a sufferer are especially high if both parents are thus affected. The resulting illness will probably *not* be the same from parent to child; thus the mother may have migraines, the father eczema and the child asthma, for example (see 'Target Organs' later in this chapter).

3 Have you ever had asthma, hay fever, chronic rhinitis, colitis, migraine, 'digestive troubles', an irritable bowel, a spastic colon or periodic depression? These questions are included because sometimes allergies are not recognised as such. The above diseases should be regarded as possible evidence of maladaptations.

4 Does your condition improve or go completely when you are away from home or work? Does it vary at weekends or when you are on holiday? A 'Yes' here is good evidence that your troubles have a basis in environmental factors. If at times you are completely well, it rather proves the point: deep down you are as normal as anyone else. There is *nothing wrong* with your body; it's just that something is harming you. Be patient, and we'll find out what it is.

SYMPTOMS

A list of symptoms follows which you can fill out, as it applies to you, by the simple expedient of ticking the appropriate box.

There can be other reasons for these symptoms – none of them are exclusive to ecology – but the ones shown in bold type are almost invariably allergy-related. In my experience, the more of these symptoms you suffer from the more certain it is that you have an allergy-based illness. Each one is selected as representative of those that I and my colleagues encounter frequently. The table is grouped into similarities to help you organise your thoughts. In general, you should concentrate on the last twelve months if you have been continuously ill in that period. You may then take a wider view and consider which symptoms have been present, on and off, *since you became ill.*

TABLE OF SYMPTOMS

	Seldom	Often	Permanent
Ocular			
Red, itchy eyes			
Sandy feeling			
Heavy eyes			
Dark rings			
Unnatural 'sparkle'			
Watering			
Blurring of vision			
Spots in view			
Flashing lights			
Double vision (comes and goes)			
'Floaters'			
Ears			
Ringing in the ears			
Itching			
Red pinna			
Earache			
Hearing loss			
Recurring infections, especially in children			
Cardiovascular			
Rapid or irregular pulse			
Palpitations, especially after eating			
Blood pressure			

	Seldom	Often	Permanent
Chest pain			
Tight chest			
Pain on exercise (angina)			
Feeling faint			
Lungs			
Tightness			
Wheezing			
Poor respiratory function			
Hyperventilation (over- breathing)			
Cough without sputum			
Throat, nose and mouth			
Metallic taste			
Mouth ulcers			
Frequent sore throats			
Catarrh (thick or watery)			
Sneezing			
Post-nasal drip			
Stuffed up			
'Sinusitis'			
Stiffness of throat or tongue			
Gastro-intestinal			
Nausea, vomiting			
Belching			
Dyspepsia (indigestion, not all the time)			
Abdominal bloating			
Flatulence			
Abdominal distress			
Pain in the stomach			
Diarrhoea			
Constipation			
Variability of bowel function			
'Stomach rumbling'			
Hunger pangs			
Acidity			
Skin			
Eczema			
Rash (not eczema)			
Itching			

	Seldom	Often	Permanent
Blotches			
Urticaria (hives)			
Excessive sweating			
Chilblains			
Musculo-skeletal			
Swollen, painful joints			
Aching muscles			
Stiffness			
Cramps			
'Fibrositis'			
'Rheumatism'			
Muscle spasms			
Tremors (shaking, especially on waking)			
Pseudo-paralysis			
Genito-urinary system			
Menstrual difficulties			
Frequency of urination			
Bed-wetting			
Burning urination			
Pressure			
Genital itch			
Urgency			
Headache			
Migraine			
'Sick headaches'			
Pressure			
Throbbing			
Stabbing			
'Solid' feeling			
Mild or moderate headaches			
Stiff neck			
Nervous system			
Inability to think clearly			
'Dopey' feeling			
Terrible thoughts on waking			
Insomnia			
Crabby on waking			
Difficulty waking up			
Bad dreams			

	Seldom	Often	Permanent
Light headedness			
Twitching			
Memory loss			
Stammering			
Maths and spelling errors			
'Blankness'			
Delusion			
Hallucination			
Desire to injure oneself			
Convulsions			
Mental state			
Stimulated			
Silliness			
Intoxication			
Hyperactivity			
Tension			
Restlessness			
Fidgeting			
Restless legs			
Anxiety			
Panic attacks			
Irritability			
Uncontrollable rage			
Smashing-up attacks			
General speeding-up			
Depressed			
'Brain fag'			
Withdrawn			
Melancholy			
Confused			
Crying			
Lack of confidence			
Unreal			
Depersonalised			
Low mood			
Hard to classify, but definitely revealing			
Falling asleep after eating			
Sudden chills after eating			
Any abrupt change of state from well to unwell			

	Seldom	Often	Permanent
Feeling totally drained and exhausted			
Flu-like state that isn't flu			
Over- or underweight, or a history of fluctuating weight			
Occasional swelling of hands, face and abdomen			
Persistent fatigue, not helped by rest			
Vertigo			
Feeling unwell all over			

Quite a list – and probably far from complete. Patients come up with new variations all the time. It really does seem that almost any symptom you care to name could, at some time or other, be caused by allergies. If you don't recognise or understand an item from the table, don't worry: the chances are that if it means nothing to you then you don't experience it. One or two items might seem rather odd, not like symptoms at all; nevertheless they are revealing and might help us greatly in our search. For instance, the group of symptoms that imply you may not be at your best first thing in the morning (and this is so usual as to be regarded as 'normal') are probably indicative of food allergies. Why? By 8.00 a.m. most people have been without food for some twelve to fourteen hours, and in many cases that is long enough to set up withdrawal symptoms. Someone who feels bad until they have eaten breakfast – say tea and toast – who then perks up is probably addicted, that is to say allergic, to those foods.

Bloating, pains, palpitations, sudden tiredness, indeed any symptom experienced shortly after food, is likely, though not certain, to have food as its cause. Moreover, if your illness is accompanied by gastro-intestinal disturbances, such as pains, flatulence, nausea, and so on, food is very likely to be the allergy, whatever the complaint.

Another whole group of symptoms that are often ignored or glossed over are the mental manifestations. Because few doctors know what they are dealing with they tend to dismiss important clues like these as merely signs of a neurotic personality. Yet tiredness, irritability and low mood are not *normal,* no matter how common. It is a pity so many people accept this unquestioningly as their lot in life. A poor marriage, a stressful job or financial worries are often assigned to the cause of feeling unwell, and it is true that these factors can aggravate symptoms; but as anyone who has been through the Food Allergy Plan will tell you, the mere avoidance of the most harmful foods leads to a startling increase in verve, alertness, enthusiasm and willingness to cope with life's setbacks. Stress then becomes secondary: it is easy to conquer if you are feeling teriffic!

A lot of us live in a kind of mental 'fog' without recognising its existence. This is easy to understand, since for many *it never lifts*! But if you have ever had flashes, albeit briefly, of feeling young again and that the world sparkles with joy, as it did when you were a child, then that is *what you are really like.* Think about it.

Saddest of all is that many young children are compelled to grow up facing this unseen barrier to learning and maturing. Lack of concentration and forgetfulness at school can have disastrous consequences for the rest of a person's life, yet it is one of the commonest of allergy symptoms. I often see children who are struggling with emotional burdens and having great difficulties with school studies. Their diets are dreadful, but no one has suggested the real cause of the problem. Time and again the plan has sorted out their dietary liabilities and they have gone on to do very well academically, which proves to me that allergies have this markedly negative effect.

Case no. 7: Maxine's story

Possibly the best-known of our patients was a young girl whom I shall call Maxine. Her case was seized upon by the media, and she became an overnight 'star' with her name in several national newspapers. When I first interviewed her and her parents, Maxine was moody, truculent and unhappy: her school work placed her at resounding class bottom; she had few friends; she vexed her parents; but, worst of all, her teachers made no secret of their dislike for her. Finally, as if that were not enough, she suffered from terrible migraine. Things had reached crisis point when it was suggested by the head that Maxine's parents should take her to a child psychiatrist. Like many of us they had a suspicious dislike of doctors of that persuasion, but being sensible people and teachers themselves they did realise that something would have to be done. Luckily, about that time they heard about my clinic in Stockport and decided to come and see me.

To cut a long story short, we found Maxine to be allergic to a wide variety of foods, including wheat, corn, egg, tea, beef, pork and yeast. Her reaction to onion was interesting. Temper tantrums were apparently a feature of Sunday evenings, and bearing in mind the above history it is easy to understand that the parents had naturally ascribed these to a resistance to going to school next day. However, it turned out that Sunday roast *and onions* was the real culprit! Since that time I'm told that Maxine hasn't had a single headache, but the truly remarkable aspect of her recovery is the way her school work has improved beyond all recognition. She moved to the top of the class in some subjects and came very near it in several others. Lo and behold, as a student she was not dim and uncomprehending but actually very bright!

Judging by her relationships with others, Maxine became a new person, garrulous and extrovert, making contacts easily. She began to bring friends home and no longer frightened them off with her wild behaviour. Teachers recognised the improvement, and this time a letter from the head, instead of complaining was full of pleasant surprise and inquired what might be the cause of the change.

The flood of calls and letters we received after Maxine's story was publicised revealed that, all too sadly, her case was far from unique. A great many anxious parents whose children have similar problems are at their wits' end, wondering what to do. The tragedy of it is that the steps needed are so very simple: a few days on the diet given in the next chapter is all it would take for most of such children to recover and begin to behave normally; for the rest, advice given later in the book would provide a remedy.

The effect of poor eating on our future generations is quite devastating. The harm it does tends to be self-perpetuating. *All* parents should study this book and its implications; teachers too.

TARGET ORGANS

Before we leave the subject of symptoms that may be caused by an allergy to food (or to any substance) it is important to understand *why* the effects are so many and varied. Symptoms often do not remain constant even within the same patient at different times. Variation can take place over hours, days or years, which gives rise to the myth that people, especially children, 'grow out of it'. All that usually occurs is that one form of disease is substituted for another. Thus an individual may in infancy suffer from eczema and lose the skin rash after a few years, but then shortly afterwards starts suffering from asthma. In the teenage years this may become hay fever; and by the fourth decade it may have moved on to become arthritis, depression or migraine. Only a very careless observer would describe this as outgrowing the condition.

Reactions are not specific to certain allergens. Wheat may cause asthma in one case, indigestion in another, colitis in a third and so on. What is important is which part of the body bears the brunt of the attack. Thus we have the concept of the 'target' or 'shock' organ, and symptoms will be referred to its function. For example, if it is the bowel which is mainly affected, abdominal pain, bloating and diarrhoea may result; if it is the skin which is susceptible, rashes could be the manifestation; an attack on the lungs may cause breathlessness, a wheeze or a cough. Get the idea?

Probably the most widely affected organ is the brain and nervous system. This is hardly surprising, since we regard this as a complex and delicately balanced entity closely involved with our psyche. The results of brain attack, or 'cerebral allergy' as it is called, can be anything from fatigue and confusion to frightening full-blown dementia. I have a schizophrenic patient who is highly allergic to cheese: whenever he eats it, he begins to hear 'voices' and loses touch with reality for several days. Far commoner are the everyday feelings of drowsiness, irritability, gloom or silly euphoria (rarely correctly observed, except by a clinical ecologist).

Hyperactivity in children is mediated via the central nervous system. Dr Feingold, a famous American children's doctor, devised a diet that is partially successful in dealing with this problem through the avoidance of foods with aspirin-like

contents, colourings and chemicals (see Chapter 11). Without
naming it as such he had made a beginning in recognising brain
allergies in children. My main criticism is that this diet simply
doesn't go far enough: no allowance is made for children who
are reactive to foods such as milk, egg, wheat and other
common offenders.

ASSESSING YOUR DIET

Now we come to look at your own diet. What exactly are you
eating? Remember: foods are not the only allergens, but you
must sort out diet problems first if you are to succeed at all. Go
through the table below and tick the appropriate columns.
Foods that you never eat, or ones you consume daily, should be
easy to spot. But what do we mean by those classified as
'often'? For the purposes of this inventory I mean *twice a week
or more*. It takes food about four days to clear from the bowel,
so if you eat a substance twice weekly it is permanently inside
you and could be making you ill without you knowing.

Review your diet for the past twelve months (or since you
became ill) and mark how often you eat each type. Ignore
seasonal variations or foods that you are ony temporarily
eating more of *unless* this coincides with a period of increased
symptoms.

FOOD INVENTORY

	Never	Seldom	Often	Daily
Meats				
Beef				
Lamb				
Pork				
Chicken				
Fish				
Other				
Fruit (including fruit juices)				
Apple				
Orange				
Banana				

	Never	Seldom	Often	Daily
Grape, raisin, sultana				
Plum, peach, apricot				
Pineapple				
Melon				
Other				
Vegetables				
Peas, beans				
Carrots				
Cabbage, cauliflower, sprouts, broccoli				
Swede, turnip				
Tomato				
Lettuce				
Onion, leek, garlic				
Pepper				
Cucumber				
Other				
Dairy produce				
Milk				
Cheese				
Yoghurt				
Ice-cream				
Dessert mixes				
Butter, margarines with whey				
Other				
Cereals				
Breakfast cereal (any)				
Muesli				
Bread				
Biscuits				
Cakes				
Pastry				
Pancakes				
Pasta				
Corn (remember corn oil)				
Rice				
Oats				
Millet				
Other				
Drinks				
Tea				

	Never	Seldom	Often	Daily
Coffee				
Herb teas				
Squashes, cordials				
Cola, Fanta, etc.				
Alcohol:				
beer and lager				
wine and sherry				
spirits				
liqueurs				
Tap water				
Other				
Miscellaneous				
Nuts				
Chocolate				
Eggs				
Soya, soy products				
Canned and packet soups				
Sweets				
Tins, packets, jars				
How often, if at all, do you				
use food from tins, packets				
and jars? Don't forget:				
Stocks				
Sauces				
Chutneys				
Preserves				
Ready mixes				
Sweets				
Candies				

TWO MORE LISTS

Now, to complete this inventory make two more lists. These are personal to you. First, a list of foods you know disagree with you. Do not include things you may have been *told* are bad for you (for example, you may have heard that chocolate is bad for migraines); include only those which you have found out by actual experience make you ill when you eat them. Secondly, a list of foods you crave or would binge on if you let yourself. If that doesn't have any meaning for you, then try to think of it as a list of things you couldn't give up easily.

The first list may be quite revealing. It is amazing how many people already know that foods can make them ill and yet never realise that their diseases are so caused also. Sometimes a patient will inform me that he or she cannot eat pork because it makes him or her ill, yet daily has bacon for breakfast: the slip did not occur to that person until I pointed it out. Similar cases are milk and beef or chicken and egg (each pair comes from the same animal).

The second list contains clues to likely addictions. However, these are not necessarily the foods that are making you ill. Tea, coffee and chocolate are highly addictive substances. I try to get patients to think of them as drugs because they have true pharmacological actions on the heart, kidneys and brain. Chocolate can on occasion make people very ill and is one of the well-known triggers of migraine, *but unless you eat it regularly, more than once a week, it is not what we are looking for*. Nevertheless, put these binge foods down. Make no mistake, they can cause symptoms.

REVIEW THE LISTS

Now is the time to look over the above lists objectively. Ask yourself: what looks unnatural? Potato crisps are an occasional indulgence for most of us. But one of my patients consumed five packets of them *every day*, along with, incidentally, two chocolate bars. She had already had one nervous breakdown and was rapidly heading for another, despite heavy doses of tranquillisers. Not surprisingly, these excesses turned out to be contributing to her illness. But the point I am trying to make is that you only had to *look* at her diet to realise it was abnormal: five slices of bread a day, ten cups of coffee, two or three bananas – these are all suspicious amounts when judged objectively. Does yours reveal similar flaws? Be honest and underline foods that you are overdoing; cut them out as part of the elimination diet in the next chapter *whether specifically banned or not*.

That completes the inventory, then. Somewhere staring you in the face on these lists may be one or more foods that have been making you suffer unnecessarily for years. Keep these records: there may be valuable information buried in them, for use later on. Also, you may use the list of symptoms as an objective guide to what progress you are making. Sometimes patients feel so well they begin to forget what terrible symptoms they started out with!

The question remains: do you have food allergies? The only way to find out is to follow the next step in the Food Allergy Plan.

5

The Elimination Diet Step

This chapter and its procedure is the key to the whole success of the Food Allergy Plan. Elimination dieting, that is the avoidance of certain foods as a means of recovery, was first pioneered as a technique by an American, Dr Albert Rowe, as early as the 1920s. Many doctors have gone on since then to verify and extend his brilliant work. A classic text on this subject is *Food Allergy* by Herbert Rinkel, Théron Randolph and Michael Zeller, which dates from 1951 (see Appendix 4).

Our own Dr Richard Mackarness added a perceptive innovation, just to show we needn't leave it all to our American colleagues. He postulated that 'safe' foods would be our natural diet and set out to discover what that might be. He spoke with Dr Blake Donaldson of New York, who had spent some time visiting museums and talking to archaeologists in an effort to establish what primitive man ate. As a result he advanced what has since come to be called the Stone Age or Caveman Diet (see Appendix 4). This consists simply of foods that were eaten by man the biological animal before he became civilised, settled down and learned how to be a farmer. This very significant evolutionary step doubtless led man to the means of feeding himself more efficiently, which in turn allowed man to expand exponentially in population and so conquer his environment; but unfortunately it gave us new foods that are not well tolerated and seem to cause the bulk of food allergy problems.

The elimination plan, given below, is simply a version of this very important therapeutic diet. Basically it consists of only meat, fish, fruit and vegetables plus water, with only slight modifications.

FASTING IS THE UNDERCUT

One logical way to find out whether you have food allergies is to fast: if you stop eating and your condition clears up, there are few who would argue that food is incriminated. Surprisingly, most people feel terrific on a fast. Instead of being tired, miserable and hungry, the majority of patients report a zest and clarity of mind which they never knew or had forgotten existed. 'I could have apeared on *Mastermind*,' said one lady (meaning the TV programme). The success of fasting rests on continuing for long enough to clear the bowel of all food residues. This usually takes about four days, but varies slightly from patient to patient. Thus it is possible to predict with a fair amount of certainty that symptoms will have cleared by the morning of the fifth day. Prior to that there are several days of 'withdrawal' symptoms, the severity of which again varies from one individual to another.

The masking phenomenon depends upon a previous 'dose' of the food still being in the body at the time of the next ingestion of that same food: thus at the end of the clearing period there are no more hidden allergies – not to food, at least. This is why the patient feels better. The corollary to this is that any food now eaten will produce a marked reaction in accordance with the severity of the intolerance. It often astonishes the unlucky patient to experience the full force of an allergy to something he or she had been eating almost daily, apparently without any ill effects.

We use this uncovering of allergies to our own advantage by allowing the patient to eat foods *one at a time*, noting which are safe and which prove to be allergies. The latter are, of course, avoided. The fact that the patient is feeling well at the time of testing makes it all the easier to spot offenders.

THE FOOD ALLERGY PLAN

If you followed the explanation given above, you will have no difficulty in understanding how the plan works. In essence, it is a compromise with fasting: instead of avoiding all foods you are asked to omit only the *likely troublemakers*. The common allergy foods – a sort of 'top ten' – are wheat, corn, egg, milk, colourings and chemicals, instant coffee, cane sugar, yeast, tea and cheese. Others seem to vary according to consumption by the patient. For example, the tomato is quite a common allergen (although you would probably think it a fairly natural foodstuff), probably because it is consumed in such large quantities; we now eat winter salads, and tomatoes are very widely used in sauces and flavourings.

Avoiding these particular foods has the same effect as a fast. If the patient recovers, then these were indeed the principal allergies; also, they are now *unmasked* and capable of being tested reliably. The presence in the body of unrelated foods does not have any masking influence on a food which has been avoided long enough to clear from the bowel. Thus we reintroduce the banned foods, one at a time, and note which ones cause symptoms. As before, these must be avoided. If recovery is only partial, it could be due to the fact that some of the allowed foods eaten during the elimination were not actually safe and were contributing to the symptoms. These in turn must be removed from the diet and tested (see Chapter 7). Alternatively, the trouble may not be due to a food at all but from an environmental chemical (see Chapter 9).

The main difference is that in elimination dieting you are asked to continue rather longer: I suggest ten to fourteen days instead of the minimum five. The correct name for this procedure is *elimination and challenge dieting*. Clinical ecologists have at their disposal a number of more advanced methods of testing, but this one still remains the mainstay of investigation into food and other allergies. All the cases you read about in Chapter 1 were helped by this approach, and there are hundreds of thousands of similar cases to prove that it works. It may work for you, too: just read the instructions below and follow them carefully.

THE ELIMINATION DIET

For convenience and ease of understanding I have divided the banned groups of foods into three categories. Read through the instructions in full first and make sure you have a good grasp of what is required. The next stage is planning. Normally it requires a change of shopping habits, never mind eating habits, and you would be wise to locate suppliers of the items you need before getting started. I usually also recommend to patients that they *remove* from the house all the 'wrong' or banned foods: that way there is no temptation.

Avoid drugs By drugs I mean medicines, 'street' drugs, remedies, cures, tea, tobacco, coffee and vitamins. It is important to check with your doctor before abandoning any treatment he or she may be giving you, but do be alert to an authoritarian and unreasonable insistence that you do things his or her way: that way hasn't been working, or you probably wouldn't be reading this book. You therefore have a right to try any sensible alternative. The fact is that *very* few drugs are essential or life-saving. Insulin, thyroid hormones, epilepsy drugs, digoxin and one or two others spring to mind; the rest, such as painkillers, tranquillisers, antihistamines, antacids, sedatives, hormone replacements and the like are not strictly essential. Even the contraceptive pill, which is a steroid hormone, would be best omitted if possible. (*Caution*: if you are using other steroid drugs or creams, turn to Chapter 13 for advice.)

The acid test is: how long have you been taking this drug? If you have been on it for years and are no better, it isn't really helping. At best it can be suppressing symptoms but not actually curing them. If you are taking any drug without really knowing why it has been prescribed, find out. Get your doctor to explain. Don't be fobbed off with the usual 'You're too stupid to understand' attitude that a great many practitioners deplorably fall into (the ignorance is usually *theirs*!). If he or she is unable to sensibly defend prescribing the drug for you, don't take it. Far too many drugs are prescribed today. Many are useless or cause complications which seem not to worry the doctor but can make life unbearable for the patient. These side-effects often result in the need for *another* drug to treat them, and matters can then become very complicated. I have on occasion seen individuals taking as many as eight or nine different drugs, several of which were to counteract the problems caused by the rest. Often the patient obtains immediate relief *simply by stopping all drugs*. I firmly believe that in a number of cases the original illness disappears and that the perpetuation of the illness is brought about by the continuance of the treatment, without anyone suspecting. This credibility gap is one of the reasons medical practitioners are fast losing face in the eyes of their own patients.

This is not meant as a criticism of my medical colleagues, though I admit it does sound like carping: the point is, you can just as easily be allergic to drugs as you can to food and chemicals, so the very treatment you are receiving could be contributing to the problem. After all, there is no such thing as a harmless drug, no matter what assurances you are given. Thalidomide was given extensive tests and hailed as safe, as *especially recommended for pregnancy*! Last year approximately seventy-five people were killed by another new drug, Opren, before it was finally taken off the market.

One of the problems with medicines is that it is not just the active compounds which cause trouble, especially for the allergy patient. Tartrazine, a commonly used yellow dye, is highly allergenic and yet responsible for the colour of almost all yellow pills. Moreover, corn, a bad allergen, and other starches may be used for binding. There are numerous other ingredients, any one of which may cause a reaction, one example being Premarin. The pill contains over thirty separate ingredients, including two hormones. Such 'cocktails' have almost inevitable consequences for the acutely sensitive allergy patient.

The last, and not the least important, reason you are asked to give up drugs is that you need to know what you are like off them and away from allergens. Even if you are neither better nor worse, that is some progress: make no mistake, anyone taking drugs I regard as in danger. If you are unable to give up your medication, go ahead with the diet anyway: improvement is perfectly possible and quite probable.

Incidentally, some of the above remarks explain why I also ban vitamins. Vitamin tablets are not dangerous in the same sense that drugs are, but these tablets also usually contain a great many additive ingredients which might be allergenic.

Case no. 8: Potato allergy

A 38-year-old woman went on a vitamin enhancement programme which called for quite large doses. She rapidly became suicidal and had to stop. This was eventually traced to the niacin (B3) tablet, which was found to contain potato starch. Potato was known to have this effect, and she avoids it meticulously, but the tablets caught her out. This case, by the way, is one in the eye for those doctors who claim that patients 'imagine' their reactions to certain foods because they know they are eating them and so fake the symptoms. (Yes, I have heard this infantile criticism from someone who should know better.) This woman had no idea, until she phoned the vitamin suppliers, that she had been eating potato.

You may not be taking *large* doses of vitamins, but this case is quoted to make the point: you may unknowingly be causing symptoms by taking *any* pills. There is the question of homoeopathic remedies. It can be said with a fair amount of certainty that such remedies are not incompatible with this diet; however, the vehicle used can cause problems. The commonest of these is the simple white tablet. Known as Suc-Lac, it contains sucrose and lactose. You may recognise these as cane sugar and milk sugar, and you will readily see that these are *not* acceptable on the diet; neither is the plain white powder preparation soaked with the active ingredient, for that is also a sugar. Have a word with your homoeopath; tell him or her what you are doing. Most homoeopaths are very open to the subject of diet and nutrition. If you explain the problem, he or she should be able to provide you with a liquid to take as drops for this period.

Alcohol is included as a drug because it has marked effects on the brain and body. Remember, if you are in any doubt, that rum was once used as an anaesthetic for sailors when cutting off shattered legs. It is highly addictive, but worst of all it increases your allergy reaction to other foods also. Dr Théron Randolph, already mentioned, refers to alcoholic drinks as 'jet-propelled food allergies' – so be warned! In any case, most alcoholic drinks contain substances that you will not be allowed to take on the diet (wheat, corn and sugar for example). What I usually say to patients is this: keep off alcohol until you are well. Then you can celebrate in champagne if you like – but he prepared to take the headache as a consequence! This is not a moral pronouncement against liquor but an entirely scientific one.

It should be very obvious why tobacco is included. Cigarettes are probably the most addictive of all the common social poisons. That is because tobacco is invariably a *masked allergy*.

If you think back to when you first started smoking, the chances are that it made you quite unwell on the first few attempts (Stage 1 allergy), but you persisted and learned to tolerate it (Stage 2). Finally a condition of dependence was reached where too long a period without a dose produced withdrawal reactions (Stage 3): by then it started making you ill. But please understand this: I am not saying that unless you give up smoking this diet will not help you; it almost certainly will. Try very hard to stop, but if you cannot that is no reason to give up on your health — try the diet anyway. Those afflicted with migraine and headaches should know of one very important statistic: half of all headache sufferers who stop smoking experience a dramatic improvement in their condition. Bear this in mind when you are next dying for a puff.

Next, tea and coffee. Make no mistake, these are powerful drugs with pharmacological effects on the heart, brain and kidneys. You must avoid them. Look around you at your friends or work colleagues: you will see an astonishingly high level of consumption of these drink substances. You should easily be able to spot the real addicts: they look anxious, restless and maybe even become short-tempered if it is 'time for a brew'. As soon as they have indulged their craving they calm down again; you are observing a masked allergy. Be sure these few sentences don't also apply to you!

Substitutes are not permitted, so decaffeinated coffee is *out*. Later, when you are well, you may be able to return to this drink: it is a big improvement on untreated coffee. But you will have to remember that the chemicals used to remove the caffeine will usually contaminate the final product and *may* cause you problems. Substitutes for tea are discussed later, but all kinds of regular tea — China, Earl Grey, Formosa, Darjeeling and so on — are forbidden.

Lastly, it is important that you recognise herbal and other remedies as drugs: in fact, many plant extracts used as treatments were later found to contain quite potent drug substances, digitalis being an example. This is not to compare the toxicity of modern drugs with that of simple folk remedies, but the fact is that no one knows the ingredients of most plant preparations. They *are* drugs and — more important from your point of view — they are certainly potential allergens.

In general, if you are in doubt, omit it. This is especially true if your 'cure' has been taken for any length of time. It obviously isn't curing you in any sense of the word, though it is possibly suppressing symptoms. You could probably manage without it at least for the test period.

Omit all unhealthy foods: By that I don't just mean junk food but items which represent a high health risk and have a proportionately low food value. Tea and coffee, for example, would have fitted just as well into this category as they have *no* nutritional content. It is vital to exclude from this diet all manufactured foods, which means anything from tins, packets, bottles and jars. The reason will be clear if you read the labels. It is virtually impossible to obtain any of these commodities free from additives such as flavourings, colourants, preservatives, emulsifiers and 'enhancers'. As if that were not enough, there is also the problem of adulteration.

Substances banned on the diet may be added surreptitiously to food: for example, tinned peas usually contain sugar (as well as green dye and other chemicals), baked beans contain cornstarch, and sausages contain wheat. At least we have the advantage of new, stricter laws relating to the labelling of foodstuffs in the United Kingdom (see Appendix 2), but this doesn't help much on the diet except to tell you that you cannot eat these foods. All manufactured foods are included, not just those pre-packaged, so salami, sausage, pork pies, pâté and similar are all unsuitable. (A trifle erratically perhaps, I usually permit bacon and ham, but these are dubious items.)* You must avoid 'honeyed' and sweetened ham; these have sugar added. Corned beef may be acceptable if you can get the sugar-free kind, but unfortunately this seems hard to come by these days. Anyone who fails to show an improvement while eating these foods should consider removing them also from the diet.

Also banned are foods derived from carbohydrate sources – especially flour and sugar. This covers bread, cakes, biscuits, pastry, sweets and confectionery of all kinds, but also a great many items such as ice-cream, gravy thickeners, dessert toppings and many fast foods which employ these substances in some way or other. I actually prefer to ban *all* members of the grain family: oats, barley, rice, corn and related cereal products. This naturally covers breakfast derivatives such as

---

*Further research has shown that bacon and ham should be completely eliminated from the diet. All references to using them in this book should be ignored.

corn flakes, Rice Crispies, porridge and the like. If you find it too tough to go without all cereals, you may relax to the point of allowing yourself rice (brown, boiled only), oatmeal (with water and salt only) or rye crackers (make sure you eat only the ones containing wholemeal rye, without wheat or corn added).* You should definitely *not* eat any other cereal products, and if you improve little or not at all in the first week, then omit even these. It is impossible to underestimate the extent and frequency of allergies to grain products – take care!

Likely allergens: Lastly, we ban a group of foods simply because they show up time and time again as allergens. They tend to be badly tolerated, and I am always suspicious of them from the start. Premier amongst these offenders is milk. Dairy products, of course, include cream, yoghurt and cheese. I think it was the author Sir Richard Burton who said much to do with milk causes melancholy, so its propensity for causing illness has clearly been known of for a very long time. Unfortunately, substitutes are not acceptable. Goat's milk (same food family) must not be used, or soya 'milk' (it contains sugar). Just grit your teeth and do without milk altogether. I'm sure some cases of 'cow's milk allergy' are in fact reactions to chemical substances which contaminate the supply, such as drugs used on the beasts (antibiotic residues from veterinary treatment are an example).

Eggs are not allowed. These are, of course, not really dairy produce, yet people sometimes think of them as such, perhaps because in most areas the milkman will deliver them if asked. They are allergenic in their own right, though not so commonly as milk and wheat. Nevertheless, egg allergy can be exquisitely sensitive: there are individuals who are unable to kiss or touch a person who has eaten or prepared an egg shortly beforehand.

Chicken is also banned. Reactions to it are quite common, perhaps because we use so many eggs in our diet. The problem is complicated further by the chemicals, such as fattening drugs, to be found in modern dressed supermarket chickens. Even so, free-range birds are not without risk, hence we omit chicken. Yet you are free to eat turkey, duck and other fowl, subject to the normal precautions against manufactured adulteration.

The citrus family are common troublemakers. Orange seems to be the worst, but it is safer to avoid them all. This includes

---

*In the USA there is no rye that does not have at least a small amount of wheat intermixed. 3% wheat is permitted in "100% seed rye".

grapefruit, lemons, limes, tangerines and similar fruit (with segments and pips).

Chocolate is, of course, forbidden, and you should take no added sugar, honey or sweeteners.

And there you just about have it: those are the precluded foods. Probably by now you are asking yourself 'What on earth is left? What *do* I eat?' Actually, all fresh meat (except chicken), fresh fish, fresh fruit (except citrus) and fresh vegetables. That's quite a lot, really. Maybe most of your favourites have gone – that's the idea! – but you won't starve.

The emphasis is on *fresh* food. Frozen cod steaks will simply not do because of the chemicals they contain, such as monosodium glutamate and other additives. This is not to say that freezing harms food: it doesn't if done properly, so your own vegetables harvested and then put in the home freezer are fine. Purchases, on the other hand, should be made at the butcher's, the fishmonger's and the greengrocer's – *not* at the supermarket.

This isn't a slimming diet, though you are almost certain to lose weight if you stick rigidly to it. Even slim people tend to lose weight to some extent, but it does stabilise out and you can always put a few pounds back on when all your allergies have been properly sorted out. You can eat *as much as you like*, the only restriction being on *what* you eat. If you feel hungry after eating, just cook the whole meal again and eat it twice.

Now we come to drinks. Drink only bottled spring water. Tap water is most unsuitable because of the large variety of chemicals it contains. Bottled water is plentiful and cheap these days; supermarkets now generally stock it. (Don't worry about the plastic bottles at this stage: the chances are that these will cause no problems.) For variety you can also obtain some of the carbonated brands, such as Perrier or Malvern. These are rather more expensive, usually purchased from off-licences. Herb teas are acceptable, and there are very many to choose from. These are an acquired taste, but it is probably worth persisting. Everyone has different favourites, and each one is liked by some and hated by others, so don't give up if the first few you try are awful; you should be able to find something you like. *Make your teas with spring water only.*

Certain fruit juices are permitted, also in moderation. These are apple, grape and pineapple, *not* orange and grapefruit. You must take care to get brands which say 'No additives'. Beware of cute manufacturers who say 'No artificial preservatives': they add what they claim to be 'natural' preservatives. This usually means lacto-fermented whey, and on a milk-free diet this is of course unacceptable. 'No added anything' is the kind of wording you should look for.

Most of my patients at the clinic become devilish label-readers: nothing gets past their hawk eyes. This is a good habit to cultivate, though it can be very depressing when you walk around the supermarket. Unfortunately, many food manufacturers are not very ethical and try to pull the wool over the eyes of the uninformed public. To take another example, you will see the wording 'No added sugar' on some food items. This often means corn syrup has been added. It is not permitted to call this product sugar, though it is a sweetener. Manufacturers make a virtue of this by labelling accordingly. If this deception were not taking place, why weren't the wordings 'Nothing added' or 'pure' used?

For the purposes of this diet, dried fruit and nuts are OK, though a word of caution is needed. Most dried fruits are treated in some way. This usually takes the form of coating with mineral oil and bleaching with sulphur dioxide. These are substances to be avoided by choice, and it is better to buy at a health food shop run by knowledgeable people who can guarantee that their goods have not been subjected to this type of adulteration (I use the word 'knowledgeable' advisedly, because it is a sad fact that many health food shops are run by individuals who haven't a clue as to what they are selling!).

Salted peanuts and other packeted nuts are useless, as they contain additives. Get dry shelled nuts only. Again, the health food shop is the best place to find these.

So that is the basic diet; now all that remains is for you to make any personal modifications. Look over your diet survey again. Try to be objective and decide if there are any foods that you eat rather a lot of which were not banned: these should also be excluded from the diet. It is hard to define what is meant by 'eating a lot of' a certain food; to some extent how you feel about it is a guide. If you are definitely keen on it and look forward to the next helping, take this as a warning of possible addiction! For example, the common potato is often eaten excessively; many people don't feel the main meal of the

day is complete without this vegetable. But do not underestimate its potential harm. I have seen a child lose virtually all
its skin due to potato, a woman who spent twenty years in
psychiatric care (including shock treatment) because of it,
asthma cases and scores of other illnesses caused or made
worse by apparently innocent helpings of mash or chips.
Similarly, every daily food should be reviewed: just why are
you eating it so repetitively? This is a question that should
always arouse suspicion. At least reduce the frequency to one
day in four as a safety precaution if you can't make up your
mind whether or not to omit it altogether.

And there we have it – quite a tough eating programme, isn't
it? But I doubt if it is any worse than feeling ill most of the
time. A lot of people find it is surprisingly easy after the
withdrawal phase is over. Remember, I am not suggesting that
you eat like this for the rest of your life! It is a test designed to
last about fourteen days. At the end of that time you should be
able to draw certain conclusions. Often the results are quicker;
sometimes, especially with 'slow' diseases like arthritis and
eczema, you may need to be prepared to go on for longer.

And for it to be a valid test from the scientific point of view
you must perform it correctly. If you are slapdash about it and
get well anyway – all well and good. But if you don't really feel
any improvement, you won't know whether it is because you
are not sensitive to the common food allergens or because you
failed to carry out the test as described. It is no good cheating
'just a little'. This is not a slimming plan where you can get
away with an occasional indiscretion and still lose weight.
Allergens work against you even in very small quantities: for a
vivid illustration of this, think how minute traces of pollen in
the atmosphere make hay fever sufferers so wretched in
summer.

We are trying to clear all traces of these particular foods
from your body. Only when you are totally free of a substance
will you know if it has been upsetting you. When your bowel is
clear of it, then it can no longer be a masked allergy; you will
react on eating the food again, even if you never noticed it
before. So you have two chances to catch the culprit: firstly, if
you feel better for not eating it, that is a good clue; and
secondly, if it makes you ill again after a couple of weeks'
avoidance, that is as near to proof as you can get.

How we carry out these specific food tests is covered later in the book. In the meantime, just don't cheat – OK?

When confronted with the diet a lot of patients say to me feebly, 'What am I going to eat?' Apparently the listed meats, fruits, vegetables and fish are to them not 'real food'. Recognise that this is either a habit or addiction situation and therefore undesirable. The whole idea of this eating programme is to force you to break your eating patterns. The very fact that the thought of giving up bread, milk and tea sends cold shivers down your spine is *precisely* the reason you *ought* to be depriving yourself of these foods.

Breakfast seems to cause the most trouble. Take away cornflakes, tea and toast, and the average Anglo-Saxon hasn't a clue how to start the day! Many people turn their noses up at the suggestion of fish, meat or fruit for breakfast. Some even look at me as if I had made an obscene remark. But look, if a food is healthy at 6 p.m. it is healthy at 8 a.m. We don't usually eat haddock and chips for breakfast, but on this diet there is no reason why you should not (fish not battered, chips cooked only in sunflower oil).

Perhaps we have certain prejudices to which we would rather not admit. I once heard a man criticise a rather stuck-up middle-aged lady as belonging to the 'fur coat and kippers for breakfast set', as if going without Rice Crispies were some dreadful upper-class affectation. I didn't tell him that for years I had been putting patients on fish breakfasts to solve the problem of low blood-sugar attacks! Be a little adventurous: let your imagination run loose. Some suggestions are given at the end of this book, but choosing what you fancy is better than following anyone else's menu.

There is a very sound reason for eating a hearty breakfast, which I have just hinted at. If you eat carbohydrate, it tends to digest and dissipate quickly. This can lead to temporarily high blood sugar which is over-corrected by the body, causing it to go too low. The victim recognises this as tiredness and hunger and so is very soon eating again. Cereal and sweet things for breakfast (bread is a cereal food: wheat) set up this trap with a vengeance. The best foods to protect you from hunger pangs are fat and protein; thus for your first meal of the day liver, kidneys, chops, fish and the like are a good investment against hunger and against the desire to stray from the diet and nibble 'snacks'.

The same enjoinder applies, though less forcefully, to your other daily meals. Also, tuck in as often as you like to fruit and cold meat for your between-meals eating. Eat heartily, and *don't go hungry*. Make a virtue out of breaking your normal routine. People may laugh at your turning up at work with fruit and a bottle of spring water for lunch; but make no mistake, they will inwardly envy you and the fact that you have the guts to do something about your health. Others who continue to eat junk will be far more uncomfortable about your diet than you will!

If you experience no change on the diet you can rejoin the rest of the human race in two weeks. But if you do end up feeling wonderfully well, then you can ride all the ribbing and turn it into admiration. There is no better salve for wounds than I-told-you-so ointment!

SUMMARY

Here, then, in tabular form, is the outline of the elimination diet. No attempt is made to list all possible foods; merely the common ones. This should be enough to guide you with non-listed items.

*On the diet you are **not** allowed to have*:

Coffee
Tea
Soft drinks
Alcohol
Drugs
Cures and remedies
Vitamins
Food from tins and packets, jars or bottles (the simple rule is: if somebody labelled it, they added to it)
Sugar, honey, sweeteners
Citrus fruit (orange, grape-fruit, lemon, tangerine, etc.)
Egg
Chicken
Dairy produce: milk, cream, yoghurt, cheese etc.
Sausage, pâté, wurst
Corned beef, luncheon meat, Spam, etc.
Frozen vegetables
Dried fruit with additives (e.g. Trail Pack)
Tap water

You may have:

Beef
Pork

Lamb
Duck
Turkey
Rabbit
Fish (all kinds)
Seafood (fresh)
Apple
Banana
Pear
Melon, cantaloup
Pineapple
Grape
Any other fresh fruit except
   citrus
Pulses (peas, beans, lentils,
   etc.)
The cabbage family (cauli-
   flower, broccoli, sprouts,
   etc.)
Turnip, swede
Tomato

Potato
Lettuce
Onion
The carrot family (parsnip,
   celery, etc.)
Cucumber, courgette
Any other fresh vegetable
Herb teas (camomile, fennel,
   rosehip, rooibosch, etc.)
Fruit juices (apple, grape and
   pineapple, without
   additives)
Spring water, still or
   carbonated
Dried fruits (sultanas, raisins,
   apricots, if untreated)
Nuts
Flours such as soya, potato
   and buckwheat

So, you see, the list of allowed foods is quite long. I hope you are not still daunted at this stage, but if you are, take heart: I promise you it isn't so bad once you get started. It is an old Chinese proverb that a journey of a thousand miles begins with the first step. If you never get started, you'll never arrive.

You may be keen to begin right away; even so, it is prudent to spend a day planning menus and shopping for the right sort of eatables. It might even pay you to throw out all the bread, sweets, biscuits, handy meats and anything else that would act as a temptation if you left it in the fridge or cupboard. One suggestion is to have a large bowl of fruit standing by and where once you would eat a biscuit because of hunger take an apple or banana instead.

If someone else does the cooking for you, then of course you must explain to that person what is needed. Nothing can be more upsetting than to wait for a meal, feeling very hungry, only to find you cannot eat it when it arrives because the recipe includes some forbidden item! If the cook refuses to co-operate and you have made it clear that this diet is important to you, then indeed you have a serious problem quite apart from ill health. But the handling of human relationships is quite outside the scope of this simple book – cope as best you can.

Since for most people the diet is quite straightforward, the following chapter tells you how to proceed on the basis of the results, whether it works for you or not. But for those with special situations, such as vegetarians, those managing children on the diet, those eating out for business reasons and so on, see Chapter 12 for helpful advice.

Let me now close this chapter with a reminder about withdrawal reactions. As with a junkie coming off heroin or an alcoholic who gets the DTs, the symptoms caused by stopping something to which you are addicted can be quite severe. Patients occasionally suffer so badly they have to give up working and retire to bed for a couple of days. It can be like this, but fortunately this extreme is rather rare: most people experience nothing more than a headache, tiredness and a disagreeable manner with friends and relations. It *can* be a trying few days, and you must warn them it might happen or you will find yourself in conflict. It is especially important to be sympathetic with children in this phase: they are not being naughty as you might think, and to punish bad behaviour would only add to the distress.

The point to remember is that if you do feel something out of the ordinary it is good news, so to speak: it means we have hit a bull's-eye somewhere. One or more of the foods you have ceased to eat was an allergen, and you are going to be correspondingly better in the long run. If that isn't comfort enough, then bear in mind that it will all clear up in a few days. Since it takes about four days to empty the bowel it is possible to predict that many cases, though not all, will wake up feeling refreshed and well on the morning of the fifth day. Patients are often startled by how accurate this is. Even if you vary by having symptoms which persist longer, your deliverance will come, so do persist.

The only exception to this last remark is the occasional individual who gets worse due to being allergic to something eaten on the diet – fruit, for example. Again, this is rare and not a reason to give up when the going gets hard. Only if you are still feeling worse after ten or more days should you suspect you might be in this category. The way to deal with the problem is explained later (see Chapter 7).

Pronounced withdrawal reactions I usually treat by recommending a mild laxative such as Epsom salts or magnesia. The idea is that the sooner your bowel clears, the sooner you will feel better. If the reactions are very severe you probably won't feel like eating at all, and it is often a good idea to simply cancel all your engagements, relax with a good book and switch to a fast. This invariably cuts short the suffering.*

Whatever happens, it is a good idea to remember that since food started it you will be able to sort it out using the information in this book.

Now that's enough of the preliminaries. Have a go and see what happens. *Bon appétit!*

---

*Clinical research has shown that, since the bowel does not always spontaneously empty during a fast, emptying the bowel with saline enemas before a fast is advisable.

6

What to do if the Diet Succeeds

Perhaps it would be worth while pointing out what is meant by success in the elimination step. Obviously, if all your symptoms have cleared up and you feel *wonderful*, you will have no difficulty in making up your mind that you have achieved a great deal – congratulations! But what if you have made only a partial recovery: some of your symptoms are lessened, some have perhaps disappeared, and others remain unchanged? This is quite a common occurrence, and you should not be despondent: there are several more steps to go through after the preliminary diet which may bring further gains or possibly lead you all the way to a cure. What you have proved is that your illness has an allergy basis. For many people this will be the first sign of progress in years, and, of course, a degree of success. What follows is an attempt to build on this initial information.

Compare yourself with the list of symptoms you ticked off in the inventory: how are you now? With hindsight, you may realise that you are much better than you thought: it is only natural to forget unpleasant feelings when they are gone. Occasionally friends will make helpful comments such as 'You look wonderful. What have you been doing?' If you are *definitely* no better (or worse), the next chapter is for you; but read the rest of this one first.

SAFE VERSUS UNSAFE FOODS

Remember that the foods chosen for the elimination diet are only *relatively* safe: it is perfectly possible that you may still be reacting to one or more of them. If that is the case, you can hardly expect to feel 100 per cent at this stage. There is no such thing as a completely safe food: I have had patients experience violent reactions to such innocent-seeming everyday foods as lettuce, carrot and onion. The masking phenomenon allows them to go undetected indefinitely unless you apply the testing procedure given in this chapter. Then there can be no doubt as to the effects, as the startled victims discovered.

To feel fully well it may be necessary to avoid *all* the foods to which you are allergic at the same time. This may explain why you are still having some symptoms. The next chapter explains how to trace foods that you may still be eating but which are allergenic.

YOU FEEL WELL

If you have recovered completely, then this is the easiest part of the book for you. Basically, what is required next is to identify those foods which were making you ill. We know there were several from the fact that you now feel better.

Incidentally, allergies rarely come singly. Many patients, I find, mistakenly expect to find one big troublemaker and that all the rest will be fine. This is not so: if you have developed one intolerance, you will almost certainly have several. Harris Hosen, one of the father-figures among American allergists, showed in a study of fifty consecutive patients that the average number of food allergies was between nine and ten per patient, though some had as many as twenty-five. My own experience accords with this. How do we now pinpoint the correct foods? To do this you must eat each item under test conditions and see what happens. Those which cause symptoms are allergies and should be avoided. Any that appear harmless may be returned to your diet and continued with, as before.

Of course, like many patients, you may be feeling so much better that you don't want to hurry to change anything; you would rather not carry out any testing for the present. That is understandable and perfectly in order. Just continue as you are, following the guidelines of the elimination diet and enjoying your newfound sense of well-being. When you are ready to proceed, follow the instructions given below. Some people are happy to stay on the diet permanently and, far from coming to any harm, remain in better health than ever before. This is only natural if we believe, as I do, that it is man's correct diet. If it suits you to do this, go ahead. For information about supplements see Appendix 6.

PATIENCE IS NEEDED

Most of you, as I know from experience, probably can't wait to get off the diet no matter how much good it has done you. If you find it tedious and restricting, this is understandable. Yet a word of caution may be needed: the foods you miss the most and are so anxious to start eating again are very likely to be the ones that were making you ill in the first place. Don't forget that addiction and subsequent cravings are strong indicators of an allergy or maladaptation. You might be lucky in this respect; there are no hard and fast rules. But be warned: it will pay you to keep a tight rein on any residual longings you may have. You must dismiss from your mind the notion that now it is all over you can simply go back to eating as you did before: something has to change, otherwise you will quickly become ill again. That 'something' is usually favourite foods eaten to excess. Such foods will in fact be reintroduced for testing *last of all*.

The correct thing to do is to start with what are probably harmless foods. Each new substance is tested carefully for safety, and those which cause symptoms must be rejected. Also, you must discontinue tests until the reaction has cleared up. This may be very inconvenient, so if you are in a hurry there is all the more reason to proceed slowly. Milk and wheat (bread) are the most missed foods and, not by chance, they are in general the worst allergens. It is better to start with items such as chicken and orange first. These are rather less likely to provoke illness, and so there is more probability of expanding your diet without ill-effect.

WARNING

The symptoms experienced when testing a food can be quite severe. It is unlikely that you will come to any actual harm, but at times you may need courage and determination to go through with this procedure. It always comes as a surprise to patients when they realise what a bad effect a food causes, yet they had eaten it every day formerly without even suspecting it. This is because of the unmasking phenomenon. If you eat a food often enough, it will be permanently within your bowel. It is already in your body when you eat it again, so logically there is no reason for a response. Your body has learned to cope with the offending substance: it has *adapted*.

Only when your alimentary canal is completely clear of that food is it unmasked: you now have no protection and will be hit with the full force of the allergy. Do not continue to eat the food: the reaction will disappear as soon as your bowel is once again cleared of it. This may take a few days. You will see at once the wisdom of leaving the 'probables' until last.

HOW TO TEST A FOOD

There is no infallible way of testing foods for allergenicity. The procedure given below is about as accurate as you can get and is a combination of methods pioneered by the American ecologists Herbert Rinkel and Arthur Coca plus my own recommendations. Follow it exactly and there will be very little chance of an allergy food slipping back into your diet by mistake.

If on testing you have a positive reaction, this is almost proof. Unusual false reactions may occur, but these can be sorted out later. Even then a reaction has *some* meaning; it might be that the method of storage or preparation induced some allergy capacity to the food which was otherwise innocent. If that is the case, then there is something useful for you to investigate anyway. Negative reactions are not so definite; nevertheless, you must make some assumptions, until proved wrong. Consider a food that doesn't react as safe. If you come unstuck, just go back over the ground and test again.

PROCEDURE FOR INDIVIDUAL FOOD CHALLENGE TESTS

1 Test a food or drink only on a day when you feel well It is no use testing food unless you are able to notice a reaction. If you are suffering from, say, a headache that day, how will you know if your test food causes headaches? True, it might make the one you've got worse. But that is too risky and, having come this far by care and diligence, why cut corners? Wait for a better day.

2 Test only at lunchtime I realise that this can be difficult with children who go to school, but there is a good reason for choosing this meal instead of others. It isn't always easy to tell first thing in the morning whether the day is a good or a bad one for you, but by lunchtime you should know for sure either way. Avoid testing at breakfast unless you feel bright and sparkling (some people *are* like that at the start of the day, believe it or not!).

Testing at your evening meal is not wise: most symptoms come on in the first few hours, and you might have a reaction in the night when you are asleep and miss it. This could spare you a little discomfort, but you may be misled as to the results of the test and become confused.

3 Eat only the food you are testing Take a reasonable portion, for example two apples, half a pint of milk or two slices of bread (no butter). Sea salt may be used if needed; not table salt. Spring water is allowed – nothing else.

It is important, if you have a reaction, to be quite sure that the test food caused it. You cannot have this degree of assurance if several items were eaten at one sitting. If you eat just the one food and within a few hours feel ill, then the cause must have been that food, or not a food at all.

4 Eat it raw or prepared very simply Cooking can alter the allergenicity of food, thus well-done beef usually has more adverse effect than the same joint or cut when underdone. Minced food is also more likely to react: breaking it up speeds digestion and in effect increases the absorption.

5 If you have no observable reaction during the afternoon, include more of the test food with your evening meal. No symptoms that day or by next morning mean that the food can generally be regarded as safe. Most reactions, luckily, take place fairly quickly, often within an hour. Note that the symptom may begin fairly mildly soon after testing and only reach full force one or two days later. It is when it first comes to your attention that counts: whatever you ate just before that time is the culprit.

6 Take a pulse count You can increase the accuracy of this procedure considerably by including a simple pulse count. Arthur Coca showed in the 1950s that allergic exposures may alter the pulse rate; it was actually his wife who had first commented that her heart raced after eating certain foods. Historically, many interesting discoveries have come out of chance observations of that sort. Credit is due to Coca, of course, for having the acumen and curiosity to pursue the finding. When he wrote his simple book *The Pulse Test* (see Appendix 4) he was unaware of the masking phenomenon, as we are today. In the same way that symptoms may not be evident if the food is being consumed up to the time of the test, so the pulse may not alter because of masking. Consequently we can be even more accurate than Coca realised when he first devised the method.

The correct way to include this extra information is to take your *resting* pulse shortly before eating a test food. By 'resting' I mean sit down for at least two minutes. If you have been engaged in any strenuous exertion, allow five minutes. Count for a full minute; don't do as nurses do and count for fifteen seconds then multiply by four, as for our purposes that isn't accurate enough. After eating the food, take a repeat pulse count at intervals of twenty, forty and sixty minutes. Keep a note of the results. (It isn't necessary for you to sit still for the whole hour, merely for a couple of minutes before the reading.) A rise *or fall* of ten or more beats per minute at any of these intervals is very strong evidence that you are allergic to the food being tested, even if you get no symptoms.

If the pulse does not rise, that doesn't mean you have no allergy. And, of course, if you do experience symptoms, *even if the pulse rate does not change,* that means you are allergic to the test item.

7 Test with organic foods if you can get them By organic foods I mean those grown in a natural way, without chemical additives or contaminants, such as crop sprays, and sold without packaging or preservatives. Apples from a neighbour's garden, if the season is right, are better than the commercial variety. A chicken that has been reared free range, without chemical additives to its feed, such as antibiotic (which is used to keep battery birds 'healthy' in unsanitary, overcrowded conditions) is better than the supermarket equivalent. Unrefined food should be used instead of pre-cooked or packaged versions.

If you can't get the ideal food, go ahead and carry out your tests anyway; use whatever you can obtain without unreasonable demand on your resources. But it is vitally important that you be alert to the implications of the contamination of commercial food sources, otherwise you will draw the wrong conclusions. For example, you may think you had a bad allergy to cabbage when in reality it was the heavy chemical residue on the leaves caused by the crop's being treated with fungicide and insecticide that made you ill. This is still perfectly valid information: it means that if you can't get cabbage free of this pollution, you must avoid it at all costs. But it might be nice to know that you *could* eat cabbage now and again, providing it comes from a safe supply! For more information on organic foods and suppliers, see the appendix on this topic.

8 Reject all dubious foods, at least for the moment If you think you reacted to a food, it is no use saying to yourself, 'I'll try again tomorrow'; by eating the food as a test you have probably masked any reaction for several days. In this interval you may eat the food and learn nothing because this does not mean it is safe for you. If it does react on the second test, soon after the first, then of course this indicates that you are allergic to it; but since this is a chancy occurrence it is better to delay for at least five clear days — longer if you are constipated.

In the meantime, get on with testing other foods. The second time around you may get a more defiinite answer, yes or no. If it remains doubtful avoid it altogether, at least for ten to twelve weeks; then try again.

As a final point, you can try testing foods prepared in different ways. Cooking, for instance, both creates and destroys allergens. If you can't take a food raw, try cooking it and repeat the test (at least five days later).

WHAT TO DO IF YOU EXPERIENCE A REACTION

As I said earlier, if you don't react to a food it is moderately sound evidence of adaptation. If you *do* react, on the other hand, it is pretty definite that you are maladapted to that food. Neither outcome is proof positive, but providing you follow the above procedure closely you should be able to rely on the results. A reaction may mean either a single symptom or that you feel quite ill with many. Regardless of how mild or severe it is, you must wait until this clears up and you feel well again before proceeding with further tests. This may be irksome, but is necessary in accordance with the first point of the procedure outlined above.

Recovery can usually be speeded up by taking a mild laxative: Epsom salts are recommended. Do not take syrups or compounds at this juncture; you have no idea what ingredients they contain. In addition, it has been demonstrated that an alkaline mixture helps. It is probable that the body fluids swing towards acidity during an adverse reaction, and this helps to correct the balance. Alka-Seltzer (*gold foil only*) may be used; or you may care to make your own formula using one part potassium bicarbonate to two parts of sodium bicarbonate. Take a dessertspoonful of the resulting mixture in half a glass of water. Few chemists nowadays stock potassium bicarbonate – most of them are given over to prepared drugs and cosmetics – but if you persist you will find one. Incidentally, don't overdo this last remedy, even though it seems to work like magic: excess alkalinity is as bad as acidity and has its own dangers and problems.

I'm sure you will recognise in the above two tried and true old-fashioned 'cures', yet they do work well. I'm convinced that many cases of passing gripes and collywobbles in years gone by were due to allergy reactions, though no one would have recognised them as such. But our ancestors did hit on the right remedy without realising how or why it worked.

DELAYED REACTIONS TO FOODS

Most allergy reactions to foods come on within two to twelve hours, in other words quite rapidly. Some are even quicker and, not infrequently, patients report an *almost instantaneous* effect when eating a food. Up to twenty-four hours is not uncommon, where for example, something eaten one morning appears to be responsible for a symptom that is present on waking the next day. Much more rarely, however, it appears that a food can cause *delayed reaction*: that is, the symptoms do not appear for over twenty-four hours, even for up to forty-eight in exceptional cases. This is especially true if the individual continues to eat that food, and I have often heard patients describe this situation as a 'build-up'. It is important to be aware of this effect when you are carrying out tests, or you may come unstuck.

Suppose you were testing milk and there was no observable reaction. 'Good,' you might think, 'I'll carry on taking milk in my diet.' This is quite proper. The next day you might test egg, and again there is no response: at the same time you are having milk. On the third day you might introduce pork and feel ill: obviously, it was the pork! Well, it may not have been if you are having a delayed reaction to milk. If this does happen to you, it can become very confusing. You may be ill again before you know where you are and have learned nothing about your allergies. What do you do? Well, the thing *not* to do is give up.

Think of delayed reactions if you do not get well rapidly after avoiding a test food that caused a return of symptoms, especially if you used the bicarbonate remedy given in the previous section. The reason could be that you are not avoiding the right food. Go back to three days *prior* to the re-onset of symptoms and eliminate all foods introduced since then. Recovery within three to four days will confirm that delayed reactions are the problem. If necessary, go back to the elimination diet exactly as given. You were well (or much better) on it, so always revert to it in a crisis or when you find yourself stuck for an understanding of what has been happening. The one helpful point in this situation is that if you are experiencing delayed-onset symptoms this tends to be consistent: in other words, you will feel like that when suffering from most or all of your allergies.

In that case, proceed with tests much more slowly: instead of trying a new food each day, introduce only one or at the most two items a week. Eat them regularly each day in substantial quantities and see if you can force a reaction. If after four days of eating something fairly intensively you feel no different, then it is indeed a safe food. You may then proceed to the next one. Don't continue to eat the safe food in abundance, by the way, otherwise you may develop an allergy to it even if you don't have one at the time of testing: moderation is the key to food indulgence and staying healthy (see Chapter 10).

WHAT TO DO IF NO FOOD REACTS ON TESTING

Even more rarely, it may happen that nothing seems to react when you perform tests. This is puzzling because, having felt better avoiding certain foods, you would naturally assume that one or more of them wasn't suiting you. This is a logical deduction and one that remains quite valid.

There are two main factors which may be contributing to this anomaly. Firstly, the avoidance of an allergen, even for as short a period as two weeks, can reduce the fierceness of the sensitivity to a point where a single test dose, or even a series of meals containing the food, becomes insufficient to provoke a response form the body. In order to understand this better it is necessary to know something about fixed and cyclical allergies.

Fixed allergies As the name suggests, these are unchanging. No matter how long the food is avoided, the response will remain the same. It is a lifelong affliction, but fortunately this is the comparatively rare type.

Cyclical allergies These are more common. Basically, sensitivity to food (or chemical) is a function of the frequency with which it is eaten (or encountered). The more you come into contact with the substance, the worse the reaction gets; the less contact you have with it, meaning in terms of *frequency* rather than quantity, the more the sensitivity will subside. Complete avoidance of the substance may mean that ultimately there is no reaction to it at all. Nevertheless, the *potential* remains: in the case of an offending food, if it is again eaten often, the allergy will flare up. It is rather like a fire which will die down to glowing embers but which if fuel is thrown on it will burst into flame once more. Cyclical allergies may become fixed, but the fixed type, by definition, does not change.

This phenomenon of cycles was first noticed by Herbert Rinkel, who used it to devise rotation diets whereby the patient ate a given food only at set intervals infrequent enough to prevent the build-up of a cyclical allergy. Theron Randolph of Chicago considers that an allergy should not be designated 'fixed' unless after two years' *strict* abstinence from it the food still shows a propensity to create symptoms. It is possible that through avoidance of an allergen it will settle down in as few as ten to fourteen days. Thus testing it after such an interval may give the impression it is a harmless food whereas in fact it was one of the causes of the initial illness. Nevertheless it must be emphasised that re-adaptation is rarely so rapid: several months are normally required.

The second reason you may be confounded by an apparent absence of reaction foods is due to the summation of effects. It is possible that none of your maladaptations are serious enough to cause problems individually; only when you eat several of the foods in question concurrently does the inherent allergy potential become magnified and start to take effect. As with drugs when administered together, it is possible that the combined effect of two is more than twice the effect of each singly, perhaps many times more. This is called potentiation. You may have heard that a combination of alcohol and barbiturates can be fatal even in modest doses. This is a poor example because it comes from the world of garish murder stories and television 'thrillers', but it happens to be quite valid. It is an instance of potentiation, and allergies may behave in the same way.

I sometimes use the example of an apocryphal individual allergic to cats, dust, chocolate and milk. All may be well until one day he drinks a chocolate milk shake and strokes a cat in the attic: at that moment all four allergies come into play, and he sneezes. It would be careless to say he was allergic to the cat, though that may be all he is conscious of that is different. But without the milk there may have been no sneezing. If he tested himself with the chocolate, milk or dust, nothing would appear untoward. In general he has no symptoms, but next time he strokes the cat nothing happens and this might be puzzling.

Another day he has a glass of milk and a bar of chocolate quite close together and develops a runny nose. But there is no cat in sight, and now he doesn't know what is wrong; he hasn't heard of food allergies anyway, and thinks he's getting a cold! It is only when all the allergens occur together that sneezing occurs. So it is with food. You may observe no particular reaction on performing individual challenge tests, yet slowly you deteriorate and revert to your original condition. This is because moderate food allergies are potentiating one another.

If you suspect this situation, then go back to the elimination diet until you feel well. Then proceed as for delayed reaction testing, allowing several days between each new food. As soon as you begin to feel less than optimum, suspect the last combination. Say you introduced bread the first week, egg last week and milk this week and that you are now noticing something is wrong. Suspect the egg/milk combination. Instead of stopping the milk, stop the egg. If it clears up, it means that egg and milk together don't agree. Obviously, milk is tolerated – you got well again while still drinking it. Egg alone was also OK because you ate it for a whole week with no ill effect. (In this example, if you *didn't* recover by stopping egg I'm sure you can deduce that either milk *must* have been the culprit or the culprit is not a food allergy at all.)

By applying the above principles you may be able to work out several combinations of foods that don't suit you; simply avoid them. Nevertheless you should study Chapter 10 with particular reference to the section on rotation diets as you will almost certainly need one of these.

A FOOD AND ACTIVITIES DIARY

Throughout this plan it is a good idea to keep careful records. One type of record that will be very helpful we call the food and activities diary. At times this will help you to work out what has been happening to you, and it may also reveal useful pointers to allergens if you know what to look for. Take an ordinary exercise book and divide the pages in half with a vertical line. Date each page, and in the left-hand column write down everything you ate and also any important activities. Foods should be listed by meal and the time of the meal entered also; include details of how it was cooked. Activities recorded would not include such intricate details as 'Tied my tie' but major items such as 'Travelled to work', 'Waxed the car', 'Visited supermarket', and so on. Again, keep notes of the time factor.

On the right-hand side of the line write down any changes in your condition. If a symptom starts up, jot it down with the time. It may also be important to note when a symptom disappears. Now you will see the value of keeping a note of times. If, say, a headache appears at about 2.00 p.m. you would notice that lunch was at 1.15 p.m., and the foods included in that meal immediately become suspect. On the other hand, if the headache started at 1.05 p.m. you would ignore lunch and concentrate more closely on breakfast. Yet as you will see in Chapter 9 chemicals may also be responsible for symptoms. So if, in the example above, records showed that you flea-sprayed the cat at about eleven, this act, too, must be included in your suspicions.

The diary will do a great deal to help pinpoint likely troublemakers. For instance, if you were fairly certain which meal was to blame, the most likely food in that meal would be one which you had not eaten for at least four days. This would mean it was unmasked at the time of eating – get the idea?

Cultivate the diary. Keep it with you wherever you travel and make sure it is up to date: it can be very disconcerting to have a reaction and find you cannot remember what you ate because it wasn't written down at the time. This isn't meant to make you paranoid about your allergies, by the way – just keep everything in perspective. It can be useful to keep up the diary indefinitely if you are constantly in difficulty, but for most people it is a temporary *tool*, simply a means of getting well.

HOW LONG DO I AVOID ALLERGY FOODS?

Once cyclical allergies have been explained, most patients realise that it is not necessary to stay off allergy foods permanently. After a due interval some of these foods will be found adapted to once again and be easily tolerated in the diet provided they are taken in moderation. As with so many things, it depends on the individual case. If you make a rapid and thorough recovery you may be in such good shape that you are able to try out the implicated foods within two to three months. But for most people this would be far too soon; six months is a safer interval. In any case, no food should be returned to your diet without being subjected to the rigorous procedure of challenge testing outlined earlier in this chapter. Even then, if you seem inexplicably worse off, remove the latest food addition at once; do not continue eating a food that causes you to feel even slightly less than optimum.

Be patient and you will be rewarded. Allergies don't disappear overnight, and it will almost certainly take a long time. But if you tackle the problem sensibly you *may* be able to return to eating some of your favourite foods. Just never lose sight of the fact that these once made you ill and can do so again.

STAYING WELL

Once you have travelled this far you should be very pleased. By now I expect you will be feeling much better, if not completely well, and have a catalogue of foods that disagree with you. You may already know far more about your *personal* state of health than anyone else could, including your own doctor (unless he or she happens to be a clinical ecologist).

If success is not yet complete, the next chapter contains information which may pave the way to it. Also, remember there are causes for disorder other than food allergies (chemical intolerance for one, and although Chapter 9 covers this topic briefly, the full facts are so diverse and all-embracing that full details will have to wait for a later book). Read also Chapter 13 (on hypoglycaemia) and Appendix 5 (on *Candida* infection), which may apply to you.

If you feel fine, now would be a good time to consider vitamin and mineral supplements to build up your defences. As I said earlier in the book, allergies may well be due to deficiencies of these vital substances since they act as enzyme precursors. Appendix 6 deals briefly with nutritional extras.

SUMMARY

- If you felt partially or wholly better on the elimination diet, there were important allergens amongst the foods you gave up.
- To find out which ones, reintroduce them one at a time and see which ones provoke a return of symptoms.
- Avoid these foods and stay well.
- Alternatively, you may want to wait for a few months and then try the foods again. Cyclical allergies die down with avoidance; fixed allergies do not.
- From then on follow the procedure for testing and any food which passes may be allowed *cautiously* back into your diet. Never over-indulge in a food which has once caused a reaction.
- If you start to feel worse, you have recommenced eating an allergy food that you shouldn't have. Simplify your diet until you feel well and proceed cautiously with the reintroduction of foods.
- Staying well is not the same as getting well, and you are referred to Chapter 10.
- Vitamins and minerals help in the fight against allergies. Even wholefoods may be deficient in these substances, so consider supplements.

7

What to do if the Diet Fails

If you feel no different on the diet, or perhaps even feel worse, do not at this stage assume you have no food allergies; in fact, if you feel *worse*, that might be good evidence that you do. The probability is that you are eating much more of an allowed food which disagrees with you. No food is absolutely safe. If, for example, you are allergic to certain meats or fruit, then you are hardly likely to feel well on the exclusion diet! Fortunately, few people feel worse on the diet; but if it happens this can yield useful information. How to proceed in that event is described below. If you are already aware of an item that you are consuming heavily, suspect that item and proceed immediately to the modified test procedure a few pages hence. If nothing seems obvious, keeping a food diary for a few days (as directed at the end of the previous chapter) should yield plenty of suspicious candidates for testing.

As stated earlier, one prime culprit I find from my practice is the potato. It is a staple that is consumed heavily, daily in most British people's diets, and so, not surprisingly, quite a common allergy. When patients are prevented from eating their 'normal' quota of bread, cakes and carbohydrate 'fillers' as they tend to be christened, potato becomes the only available substitute, and it is not unusual to find people eating it twice, even three times a day while on the elimination programme.

It is far from being harmless: I have seen several very severe cases of potato intolerance. Over the years I have come to accord it the respect due to an enemy. The first time I was made strongly aware of its potential was in the case of a little boy of eighteen months. He came to me in a pitiful state, howling, puffed out like a bladder full of water and covered in eczema.

His skin was cracked and weeping, looking like a split tomato. He was being smeared with ointments which added to the mess and ooze, and had only just come out of hospital, apparently discharged because nothing else could be done for him. His frantic parents thought he was going to die.

A careful diet survey of the kind you did in Chapter 4 revealed only one daily food, which was potato, so I had his parents eliminate it completely and rotate the rest of his foods (see Chapter 10). Within a week his skin had closed off and ceased weeping, he no longer cried, and he had passed a great deal of fluid via kidneys and bladder and returned to normal size and weight. A month later he was virtually normal, but even then his parents were not quite convinced. They told me, chagrined, that they had given him one meal of potato chips. That same night he had scratched himself till he bled, and the next morning he was covered in sores. They did not repeat this experiment. Since then there have been many occasions when I have found lives blighted by this vegetable.

But of course any food could be as dramatic in its effects. The result really lies with the individual patient's susceptibility and the target or shock organs involved. All you can infer if you feel worse on the diet is that one of your worst allergens is probably among the allowed foods.

YOU FELT NO DIFFERENT

When correctly chosen for the elimination diet, about seven out of ten cases improve, one feels worse and the other two feel no change whatsoever. The first point to check, if you are in the latter category, is: do you qualify? The self-inventory in Chapter 4 is designed to establish this. Perhaps you should look over the points again. The more positive answers you give to the table of symptoms, the more certain it is that we are dealing with an allergy or intolerance. It may not be food: chemicals and inhaled allergens can have an equally devastating effect (see Chapter 9). In the meantime, finish the review given below.

DID YOU CARRY OUT THE DIET CORRECTLY?

This is a vital point: if you didn't do it exactly as written you may have denied yourself the beneficial result. This is not like a slimming plan in which you can eat just a teeny piece of chocolate cake and still lose weight. You must remember what we are trying to do, and that is clear your bowel *completely* of the suspect foods. If after four days of being careful you then slip up and eat something forbidden, it means that we have to wait another four or five days for it to clear. In the meantime you may make no recovery, and we shall learn nothing. If you lapse again, we'll get nowhere.

So — did you stick to it *rigidly*? This isn't a moral or character-building point but a very practical one. Allergies can cause effects in the most minute quantities; if you doubt that, think what infinitesimal traces of pollen do to hay fever sufferers in the summer. A mouthful of food is a vastly greater quantity in proportion, so you must be very strict with yourself.

One of my patients is so sensitive to tomatoes that he cannot enter a room where they are being cut up without having an immediate asthma attack (incidentally, he was eating them regularly when we commenced the plan but the severity of the condition was completely masked). There are cases of individuals who cannot touch an egg, or even handle an object which has contained egg, without getting a skin eruption. These are, needless to say, extremes. I am only making the point that quantity is unimportant, therefore lapses may defeat the whole plan.

It does happen that certain individuals feel better even if they restrict foods carelessly and make mistakes. But they are lucky; you mustn't count on chance. It is more scientific to *make* things work in your favour. Nothing could be more disappointing than to struggle through two weeks of deprivation only to find you did not get well because of carelessness. You might even be misled into thinking that you were not a food allergy case and miss the very cure that you are seeking. If you have not followed the diet correctly you have little choice other than to start again and follow it as written for *at least seven more days* before making up your mind as to the result. If you *then* feel no better, you may assume that the diet did not help and proceed as given in this chapter.

TESTING THE BANNED FOODS

Just because you feel no better on the elimination step does not mean that you cannot be allergic to any of the banned foods. This is because of the effect that Dr Doris Rapp describes as the 'eight nails in the shoe syndrome' (see Chapter 2). It is the same with allergies: sometimes it helps enormously to stop or reduce the number of allergens you are eating or breathing, yet you may feel no better at all because of the remaining maladaptations. Thus on the elimination diet you may consume large amounts of meat and be made ill, which would offset the benefits derived from stopping milk, wheat and coffee even though these were also potent allergens.

Accordingly, we would like to test the eliminated foods before permitting them back into your diet. Because of the stipulation that you must feel well on a day you test, if your complaint is continuous it may not be possible at this stage to reintroduce any items. We must take further steps to produce some improvement at least, as given below. If your condition is cyclical – coming and going so that there are several days at a time when nothing seems to be wrong – you can carry out the test procedures during a remission phase. You may be pleasantly surprised to detect an unsuspected allergen that way and, naturally, you would be better to avoid that food, whilst working through the remainder of the procedure in this chapter.

MODIFIED TEST PROCEDURE

We must now try to detect any hidden allergies among the 'allowed' foods of the elimination diet. Set yourself a programme of testing each one in turn. It is logical to start with those you consume most of or, more exactly, consume most often: over-indulged foods are always prime suspects. The test procedure outlined in Chapter 6 is quite valid, *with one important modification*: because of the masking effect you must strictly avoid a food to be tested for a minimum of four clear days, testing on the fifth day. If you seem constipated, test on the sixth or seventh day to be certain it is voided from the bowel. If you feel better avoiding a food, this is persuasive evidence that you may be allergic to it. If on your test dose symptoms return, this becomes almost a certainty.

The problem arises when you feel no better for avoiding a food. Trying to test when you already have symptoms is always chancy, but it is still worth doing and results can be obtained: a positive reaction is, after all, still positive. It is only when you are vague or feel no different that a food which shouldn't can slip through the net. The thing to do is to mark your notebook to that effect so that you can always come back to the food in question and test it again, supposing that we arrive at a stage where symptoms are either reduced or have disappeared completely.

KEEP GOOD RECORDS

I have said before that keeping accurate notes can be of inestimable help in this detective work. To make it easier for you to work rapidly through your present diet, testing each item and making sure each one is allowed the proper clearing interval, you are advised to draw up a chart as shown below. This will allow you to telescope the tests into the shortest possible period of time. Along the top of each column you can designate the day, either by 'Day 1, 2, 3' and so on or by giving

Day	1	2	3	4	5	6
Stop	pork	oats	beef	pea	apple	tea
Test					pork	oat
Reaction					−	−

Day	7	8	9	10	11	12
Stop	wheat	etc.				
Test	beef	pea	apple	tea	wheat	etc.
Reaction	headache	−	rash	−	−	

the date of the day in the month, such as '13th, 14th, 15th' and so on. Begin by omitting the first food on Day 1 and enter that in the top box for that day. When it is due for testing write its name in the centre box for that day and enter any reaction below, in the space provided. The examples given should make this quite clear.

At any point while carrying out these tests you may begin to feel better. It may not happen all at once – sometimes improvement comes slowly – but it is important that at the first sign of recovery you keep doing *exactly* what you are doing. Don't change your diet at all, at least for some time or until the improvement ceases; then go back to testing as before. But do realise that you must have dropped from your diet a major allergen. Make sure you know from your records what it was – and keep off it!

OMITTING GROUPS OF FOODS

Dr Jean Monro, one of Britain's foremost clinical ecologists, programmes her patients to omit groups of foods at a time. If up to this point nothing else has succeeded, you can try doing the same thing for yourself, as outlined below.

MEAT-FREE

Not everyone feels much better as a vegetarian, but you have only to read the success stories of some people who have adopted this lifestyle to realise that it suits quite a number. We can deduce that these people must have been allergic to meat in some form or other. Unfortunately, many more people are allergic to grains and dairy produce than to meat. This is sometimes hard to get across to vegetarians, who tend to be enthusiastic campaigners. It means, in effect, that fewer people are suited to vegetarianism than are made ill by it. This is an overall view, which does not take into account individual cases. Where vegetarianism *does* help is that it tends to be part and parcel of a movement towards wholefoods and away from manufactured and 'junk' food. Inevitably this is associated with increased health and vitality.

To illustrate the point I am making, let me describe the case of a young woman in her late twenties who came to see me because of asthma. At college she had become interested in health foods, healing and the occult; she then decided to be a vegetarian. For a long time this apparently suited her and harmonised well with the way of life she and her friends led. However, while engaged in full-time study she began to notice that her mental faculties were not as good as she knew them to be. Things got worse. She became drowsy and apathetic; her brain wouldn't clear in the morning and she tended to forget what she was doing, even where she was at times. As the listlessness grew worse, she became unable to attend college and at one stage ended up in a zombie-like trance which lasted many weeks. She would lie in bed, out of touch with reality and to the despair of her friends, rising only occasionally to eat a little food, perform her natural functions and go back to bed. This continued day after day for almost three months.

Then she had what she described as a vision of a fish and realised that it meant she should eat some. This she did, and felt a little better. That prompted her to try eating meat, and from then on she improved rapidly: within a matter of weeks she was her old self, resumed her studies and graduated successfully in the normal time.

It is remarkable – and perhaps fortuitous – that students living away from home can experience such ill health and that it can remain undetected. As it was, she had a lucky escape. It is no exaggeration to say that, like so many allergy patients, she might have ended up as a lifelong, institutional case in a psychiatric ward without anyone suspecting the real reason. Instead, a lucky change of diet cured her. All this emerged in the course of our discussions about her asthma, which she suffered from quite badly. The Food Allergy Plan was extremely successful in her case, and it became obvious that she was severely allergic to the grains. Even today, if she exceeds one slice of bread in twenty-four hours her mental condition deteriorates markedly, and a real binge drives her out of touch with her surroundings to an alarming degree. Yet for years she ate heavily of the grain family, as vegetarians often do. Undoubtedly this built up her cyclical allergy to wheat, and her excursion into meatless eating was almost a disaster.

Nevertheless, many people are made ill by meats, especially

the commercial variety which almost invariably has chemical contaminants of some kind, such as hormones and antibiotics. It is a practice with some suppliers to treat meat with agents to keep it red; niacin, also known at vitamin B3, is such a substance. That could be healthy, you might suppose, and so it could; but niacin is notorious for the side-effect it produces of a burning flush, rather like being exposed too long in the sun. If a hearty steak tends to do this to you, perhaps it is the 'harmless' vitamin pollution.

Include a two-week meat-free regime in your self-assessment programme. If there is any improvement, find out which meats by reintroducing them as before.

PULSE-FREE

The elimination diet or Stone Age diet is in effect grains-free, dairy-free and chemical-free with a few refinements, such as no sugar and stimulants. Next to these foods, the pulse family is arguably the commonest group of troublemakers. These are also called legumes (peas and beans). It should not be forgotten that peanuts (a bean, not a true nut), lentils and soya (often used as textured vegetable protein, TVP) are also members of this group, which, incidentally, is a true food family.

There are a great many biological toxins to be found in pulses, which means that most of them are poisonous. This could account for the fact that, as a family, they are not always well tolerated. You may be familiar with the fact that the red kidney bean – used in chilli con carne – is toxic until boiled. Other beans are known to be responsible for lathyrism, a paralysis common in India, and favism, a haemolytic anaemia common around the Mediterranean.

Thorough ccoking destroys most of the toxin (but not all allergenicity), and A.C. Leopold and R. Arthrey have pointed out that it is probably only since the advent of fire that man has been able to eat a number of foods, such as the pulses, which are inherently toxic. It is quite probable that primitive man's conquest of his environment began as a result of his being able to eat a much wider diet and so able to increase in terms of numbers to a degree impossible before that time. These are interesting speculations, and they put the enormous value of the discovery of fire into perspective for us. If they are true, it would mean that pulses, like cereals and dairy produce, are relatively new food substances for us and that we have not had long in which to adapt to them.

After your meat-free experiment, try two weeks pulse-free.

NUT AND PIP-FREE

Some people don't tolerate fruit very well; with others, it is nuts that are a problem. Eating fruit-free is sometimes so successful that a famous book for arthritics lays great stress on it. However, since it allows the eating of grains, a *much* commoner cause of arthritis, it is not a book I recommend. People allergic to nuts are usually astonished when they find out, it never having occurred to them that these could make anyone ill. It is worth trying a period without either. The tomato is not a fruit but actually a member of the same family as the potato; but because of its seeds, which are like pips, I use this modification of diet as a chance to avoid tomatoes for a trial period. If you consider this ubiquitous plant for a moment you will realise that we eat it a great deal, which is of course the formula for developing hidden allergies to it. In purée form it is found in a great many sauces and dishes, and it is often included in salads. With the international growing and shipping of fruit and vegetables, salads are now almost as commonplace in winter as in summer; thus the tomato is no longer seasonal and is a potential allergen of which you should take special note.

Fruit-free is particularly appropriate if you felt worse on the elimination diet. Most of us are used to a fairly sweet diet which includes cakes, desserts and the like, and if these are banned we lean heavily on fruit as sugar-containing substitutes. Happily for the majority of us, this is a very healthy alternative: such carbohydrates are much gentler on the system than the 'shock' of white sugar, refined flour and corn sweeteners, which are far from biological (see Chapter 13). You probably increased your fruit intake automatically, and if you feel worse try to eliminate it as part of the programme.

In all the above modifications it goes without saying that

after your experiment you should subject each item to the proper testing procedure before allowing it back into your diet. This is mandatory if you felt an improvement when on any step. The obvious conclusion is that one or more of the group you gave up were true allergens, and it is important to locate which one(s).

FASTING

Finally, if all else fails and you have any patience left, you can consider a fast. This will settle once and for all whether there is some other factor in your illness than allergy to food. Review your condition carefully. You have probably been through many trials and tribulations before reaching this point. You might feel like giving up: that is understandable. If you think going on is too difficult, I do urge you to make contact with a professional clinical ecology doctor: Action Against Allergy (see Appendix 3) can probably help.

If you are tired and run down and have lost too much weight, now is not the time to start a fast. Instead, give yourself a break, eat well and take a holiday if you can. Then come back to the problem. A word of warning, however: don't let solicitous busybodies depress you with too many adverse comments. Sometimes this may *make* you feel ill. There is a very powerful psychology at work here. You may be under a great deal of pressure to desist from what you are doing. For one thing, watching others diet makes food addicts feel very uncomfortable, and they may carp at you for what is really no more than a self-centred reason. Also, there is a tendency to associate weight loss with ill health, though the two are not always connected. Someone, I think rightly, said that we should all weigh the same as we did at the age of twenty-one; few of us do. The so-called 'average weights', usually quoted from insurance company statistics, include measurement of the obviously obese types. If the upper heavyweights in each height range were excluded as obviously abnormal, then the average weight would fall markedly: in other words, most of us should, ideally, weigh less than we do or less than the 'average' weights say we should.

When you are ready to try a fast, the next chapter tells you all you need to know. Eat a full diet for at least two weeks and stoke up with vitamin and mineral supplements in preparation (see Appendix 6) provided these do not disagree with you.

OTHER REASONS FOR FAILURE

There are other reasons why you may remain ill despite the diet. You may well have food allergies, but there could also be other factors which are denying you your recovery.

OTHER ILLNESSES CONCURRENT

Sometimes a medical diagnosis is missed: I regularly see patients with an obvious goitre, or abnormal urine tests, anaemia and other problems which should have been detected by the family doctor but weren't. If you think this may be the case with yourself, you can go back to your GP and ask about a more thorough check-up. He or she may feel this is unjustified: many doctors view allergy patients as freaks, refusing, regardless of their intelligence or reliability, to take them seriously. In that case you have no option but to ask for a second opinion. It is your right, and your doctor should not be offended by the request. Yet because of the limitations on the National Health Service you may need to seek this further advice privately.

Chemical allergies These may be to blame in your case, especially if you are well qualified as an 'allergy case' according to the self-inventory. This is quite a complex problem and is the subject of a book at least. Chapter 9 covers this problem for you in outline and will enable you to make a start on identifying the common sources of chemical allergy. It is often necessary to combine a dietary and chemical search in order to draw the 'eight nails in the shoe'.

Thrush infection It has recently been found that the causative organism of thrush, *Candida albicans*, is implicated in a wide variety of food and chemical intolerances. Furthermore, it appears to be toxic in its own right. Factors which may suggest the possibility are: a known infection (for example, a vaginal irritation that recurs intermittently); the long-term use of antibiotics for any reason (such as tetracycline for acne); the administration of steroid drugs; the use of the birth control pill for more than two years consecutively; and a tendency to feel worse in damp or mouldy conditions or after consuming yeast foods or sugar. If any of these apply to you, see Appendix 5 for more information.

Hypoglycaemia   Often dubbed 'the missing diagnosis', hypoglycaemia is probably even more under-diagnosed than allergies are. It means blood sugar that is too low. This affects the brain and other organs in much the same way that an allergy attack does. Similarly the symptoms can be complex and varied, and it is true to say that any symptoms an allergy can produce, so – with a few exceptions – can hypoglycaemia. Suspect this if you eat a meagre breakfast (or none), crave sweet foods and feel the need to eat often, especially on the elimination diet. It can be very difficult to separate hypoglycaemia from allergies, and sometimes the investigations are best run side by side. Chapter 13 is devoted to this topic, and you may care to advance to it before pursuing a fast.

Vitamin and mineral deficiency   It is an unpleasant truth that if you are eating foods which in effect act as poisons you will damage the mucous linings of your intestinal tract. Since these linings are essential for the proper performance of the digestive functions and the selective absorption of necessary vitamins and minerals, most food allergy patients become very deficient in proper nutrients. This becomes a self-perpetuating problem because a lack of these nutrients makes the allergy problem worse. Over a long period such deficiencies can become very serious.

The whole body depends for its proper functioning on correct and adequate nutrition; therefore it is not surprising if you feel unwell when lacking essential vitamins and minerals. You may need to take supplements early on (as a rule we defer this step until you have tracked down all your hidden allergies). Try the effects of taking extra nutrients as outlined in Appendix 6. If you experience any improvement, build on this with a much wider supplementation. In order to do this you may need to seek advice; alternatively, read one of the recommended books on the subject and work out a full programme for yourself (see Appendix 4). Note that it is no use supposing that all the essential supplies are in your food. They may well be; but if you are not absorbing them you will remain deficient. This point puts paid to the idea of a 'balanced' adequate diet. There is no such thing if your gut is not performing!

SUMMARY

If you do not progress while on the elimination diet it is logical to suspect some of the foods you are still eating.

- Did you do the diet correctly in the first place? If not, follow it again without lapses for a further seven days at least.
- If you are then no better, eliminate the 'allowed' foods one at a time for a period of not less than four clear days and test each one on the fifth day, as given in Chapter 6.
- Avoid any food which reacts. Once you start to feel better, also test the original 'banned' foods.
- Try periods of avoiding groups of foods, for example of going meat-free, pulse-free and nut-and-pip-free. If there is any improvement, test each food carefully.
- If all else fails, consider trying a fast. Give yourself a rest and prepare for it by eating plentifully and taking vitamin and mineral supplements.
- Make sure there are no other reasons for feeling unwell. Get another check-up from your doctor, or a second opinion.
- Could the problem be a chemical allergy (Chapter 9)? *Candida* (Appendix 5)? Or hypoglycaemia (Chapter 13)?
- Take vitamin and mineral supplements (see Appendix 6 for elementary advice).

8

The Fast

There are on the market a great many books on the subject of fasting. None of them seem to mention the phenomenon that the food allergy/addiction patient will encounter: withdrawal reactions. Naturally, their authors believe in the health-giving properties of a fast and go on to extol the virtues of a 'good clean-out': 'purification' is the ritual word often used. I think a great many readers must be severely disappointed and feel misled when they feel bad on a fast – and make no mistake, it is possible to feel dreadful.

Without an understanding of the withdrawal effect it is hard to interpret symptoms caused by fasting. In many cases, I feel sure, the difficulties may lead to a premature abandonment of the attempt, whereas of course the worse the symptoms due to a fast the more significant the cure – and only persistence brings this. Moreover, I have seen very little stress laid on the length of time needed for an effective fast. To read some enthusiastic proponents you would imagine that all the benefits are to be had starting the first day, yet this is rarely so. Many even speak of a three-day fast. All this misguided advice is missing the point: it takes about four days to be sure the bowel has cleared, and to fast for a shorter period means you are *not* free of all foods. Patients with a stubborn bowel may need to allow even longer. Of course, short-term fasting does work for some; I have no doubt that was the case with the authors who advise it. But they are then guilty of the all-too-common mistake of supposing that what is good for them is good for everybody – it rarely is.

So let me, as a clinical ecologist, say that the *minimum* fast advocated is four days. That means that if you feel well you can begin introducing foods on the fifth day – *not sooner*. There is of course no point in starting the test introductions until you do feel well, so you may need to go on longer. However, without expert medical superivison – and by that I mean a doctor who has had experience of managing fasts – the longest you should continue a fast is for seven days. It has its own hazards, which come into play the longer you carry on; therefore you must not prolong it needlessly.

Let us be quite clear: all we are trying to do is clear the bowel so that we may carry out food tests without the masking effect obscuring the result. We are not trying to strengthen your will-power, to 'purge the poisons' (except perhaps metaphorically) or to do anything other than that one simple thing.* The best guide to when your bowel is clear is how you feel. If your symptoms suddenly clear on or about the fifth day, that's what we want. If this has not happened by the eighth morning (unless you have been very constipated), it probably never will and you must desist. In that event it is almost proof positive that you do not have food allergies and you must look for chemical intolerances instead. Or seek the help of a skilled and qualified clinical ecologist.

PREPARATION

Responses to fasting vary enormously: some people make light of it and continue their normal work routine; others are prostrate and take to their beds for virtually the entire period. Most fall somewhere in between. You must assume a possible reaction that will prevent you being able to work and make arrangements accordingly. I feel bound to advise you to tell your own doctor what you propose to do in advance. Yet in most cases I am afraid that doing so will invite scorn and hostility, which you must be prepared for. Also, don't expect much helpful advice because most general practitioners are simply not trained in this technique; their opinions would rest only on the popular prejudices and misconceptions about food. Having said that, your doctor *is* your doctor, and if you are not prepared to do what he or she says don't go to the surgery in the first place!

---

*It helps to take a purgative rather than to rely on spontaneous clearing of the bowel. Epsom salts or a simple vegetable laxative are suitable. An enema is even better.

EAT WELL BEFOREHAND

It is a good idea to prepare for a fast with a few days of good, nutritious eating. For this reason it is not recommended that you fast following a period of severe restrictions on your food intake such as might occur while experimenting with elimination. If that applies to you, return to a full eating programme temporarily. This does not mean that junk food must be reintroduced, but simply that you should consume a proper balance of protein, carbohydrates and fat.

This advice does not conflict with the occasional need of a person who gets severe reactions on the exclusions of the eating plan to move into a fast. If the withdrawals are very bad, I usually suggest abandoning the diet and eating altogether. This usually cuts short the suffering – a process which can be further speeded up by taking Epsom salts to clear the bowel. Vitamin C (two to ten grammes a day) also appears to help, as it often does with toxic reactions. This high dosage should be curtailed as soon as symptoms begin to diminish. Don't wait for a complete recovery, as the vitamin C might itself cause a reaction. This is rare, but if I tell you that most vitamin C is manufactured synthetically from corn derivatives you will see at once why that could apply: corn is one of the commonest allergens of all.

It is also a good idea to take a few vitamins before you begin the fast. I don't think you should attach too much importance to doing so at this stage as it takes many months, or even years, to correct vitamin deficiencies. None the less I am a great believer in hedging bets, and I suggest you follow the basic formula given in Appendix 6. But do be alert to the fact that vitamin pills might contain something that doesn't suit you; if they seem to disagree with you, stop taking them and see.

USE A STEP-DOWN APPROACH

Unless you have a will of iron, you can make it easier on yourself when starting a fast by using a step-wise approach. Spend a day eating only a chosen fruit – say, grapes – and drinking spring water. Next day take only the spring water, and you will have moved into a fast fairly effortlessly. Count the grapes-only day as part of the fast, *but only proceed with food testing on the fifth day if you feel quite well.* You would not, of course, test grapes that day in case they are not voided from the bowel.

AVOID CHEMICAL EXPOSURES DURING A FAST

In my experience, people who are intolerant of foods also have a lot of trouble with chemicals. This may not apply to you, but why give yourself an unnecessarily hard time? Don't take risks. It is much more sensible when planning the fast to arrange that you will have as little exposure as possible to any noxious substance. Bad smells are a guide to what to avoid. For example, try to avoid urban traffic with its petrol fumes even if it means staying at home. See to it that no aerosol spray of any kind is used in your presence. Remove perfumes and cosmetics from the bedroom. Do not use powerful detergents, solvents, cleaners or bleach during this period.

Needless to say, you should not smoke during a fast. I repeat again: tobacco is a toxic substance and is almost universally a masked allergy among smokers. Also avoid smoky environments.

Keep away from cats, dogs, dust, pollen and mouldy environments if at all possible. If you can't avoid them completely, keep exposure to a minimum.

Paint, especially the gloss type, can be very offensive: make sure you have no contact with freshly decorated rooms. The consequences can take several days to clear up.

Finally, *avoid anything you have found by experience to be inimical to you.* 'Don't court symptoms' is the summary of this section!

ACTIVITIES DURING A FAST

Patients sometimes ask despairingly how to pass the time during a fast. Actually, there is plenty to do. The withdrawal phase can be unpleasant, but only very rarely does it necessitate the sufferer taking to his or her bed. It is much better to keep going rather than lie between the covers introverting and brooding. Bearing in mind the restrictions I have suggested in the preceding sections, it is perfectly possible to work. During my fast I kept up a busy twelve-hours-a-day routine, and there is no reason why you should not do the same unless your work is heavily physical. I have strict control of the environment at the clinic. If you have no control over your work area, or your work involves a lot of odorous chemical exposures (it ought not to since the Health and Safety at Work Act, 1974), it would be better to stay at home.

By the way, I consider it quite proper to utilise sick leave to carry out a fasting procedure. In Britain at present you can sign yourself off work on health grounds. It is quite legitimate to say you were absent due to illness because it is in fact true (though it would be better to put your main complaint on the claim form rather than write 'Fasting', which is likely to be misunderstood). It is important not to abuse these new privileges, but at the same time you are making a bona fide effort to get well, and – who knows? – in the long run it may result in less absence from work. It is probably best to avoid contact with strangers where lengthy explanations would be difficult or embarrassing. But your family and friends, who ought to support you, can be the object of a visit or companions for a number of activities; just steer clear of any hostility or scorn.

HOW TO COME OFF A FAST

So many patients tell me they have tried fasting and felt *wonderful* yet were unable to tell me which foods produced a reaction. This indicates that knowledge of the correct way to come off a fast is even more lacking than knowledge of how to carry one out properly. Obviously, some foods must have been to blame, or the fast would not have been beneficial. The *ideal* time to find out which ones is at the point of coming off the fast.

If you understand that fasting and clearing the bowel of food means that all food allergies are then *un*masked, you will see at once that after a fast is the very best time to carry out tests. To just begin eating willy-nilly again and get all your symptoms back is a waste of this valuable opportunity: all it tells you is

that you are allergic to foods, but not to which ones. The correct way to proceed is to reintroduce foods to a plan, perhaps two or three a day. Each one is eaten singly, under test conditions, and those which provoke a reaction are of course eliminated. If you are free of symptoms, this is very straight-forward to do as you should notice any deterioration in your condition quite easily.

The secret is to begin with foods which are *most unlikely* to be a problem. The target is to get you onto a few safe foods as quickly as possible. If you do get a symptom, you will have to wait until it clears up before going on to the next item to test using exactly the same food-testing method as that given earlier in the book. While this is not a disaster, it will certainly be most inconvenient: the last thing we want is for you to have to fast for several more days!

So we begin with fairly exotic items on the first day. Choose foods you wouldn't normally eat or never have. The table below offers some suggestions, but it is important that you understand you are free to pick your own menu. Add three new foods a day maximum. If a food is safe, you may repeat it again as often as you like; so, for example, if salmon is OK you may eat it at every meal along with the new test food until you get bored with it. However, as always, it is better to not be too repetitious once you have several choices available – ring the changes. From the third day onwards, test your usual foods but once again start with those that you consider relatively unlikely troublemakers (meat, fruit and vegetables). Don't risk wheat, milk, eggs or other 'bogey' foods at this stage; try to expand your available diet as far as possible before getting too adventurous.

Finally, of course, you must face up to introducing the probable villains. Remember the reactions can be surprisingly severe. Don't forget to warn your family or friends about this point in advance. If you are unlucky enough to have a bad reaction and – after all, in a way, that's what we are seeking – *keep up with the foods so far found safe*. Take the Epsom salts and bicarbonate mixture given in Chapter 6. Just stop testing new foods until you feel well again; then continue.

If you are doubtful about a particular food, do not try it again for several days, otherwise *you cannot be sure it is safe because of the masking effect*. The previous meal may mask

Suggested Schedule of Food Tests After a Fast

Days 1-4		No food
Day 5	Breakfast	Poached salmon
	Lunch	Mango (plus salmon)
	Dinner	Steamed spinach (plus salmon and mango)

Remember: if you did a grape-day step-down, do not attempt to test grape on Day 5.

Day 6	Breakfast	Baked pheasant, partridge or rabbit (+ salmon, mango, etc.)
	Lunch	Kiwi fruit
	Dinner	Steamed marrow, courgette or squash
Day 7	Breakfast	Lamb chop
	Lunch	Baked potato (do *not* eat the skin)
	Dinner	Banana

and so on . . .

any further reaction, so you must set that food aside and come back to it after a minimum of four days. If the second challenge, several days later, is still equivocal, then it is best to treat the food in question as a probable allergen and remove it from the schedule. Do not disregard minor symptoms, either; these could be significant. Continue only with foods which are demonstrated without doubt to be safe. Incidentally, you may increase the accuracy of these tests by using the pulse check as explained in Chapter 6.

It may happen that without any specific reaction you find yourself unwell again after a number of foods have been reintroduced. Stop as soon as this happens; don't just plough on with more foods. Think back to what you were eating when you were last doing fine and eat only those foods till you feel better. Then go on with a *different* set of new foods. Finally, return to the doubtful ones and sort them out as best you can. If it still isn't clear which is to blame, abandon them all for ten to twelve weeks and try again. In this way, within ten to fourteen days you should have built yourself a safe diet which you can follow without any untoward symptoms. If so, congratulate yourself: you have done very well. Patience, care and forbearance have brought you their reward: a knowledge of your health that is priceless and could not have been gained any other way.

THE HALF-FAST

If you really cannot bear the idea of a total fast, you may follow what I call a half-fast. Simply eat any one fruit and one meat of your choice for the five-day period. Lamb and pears are often chosen, but there is no special magic to them. All the above advice holds good, as for a complete fast, but it goes without saying that you will not get well if you happen to be allergic to either lamb or pears! You must simply take that chance. If you suspect that you may be, simply switch to two other unrelated foods.

IF THE FAST DOESN'T WORK

The fast may not help you. As with the elimination diet, the fact that it doesn't is no proof that you don't have food allergies; but the probability that you have diminishes close to vanishing point. Yet it could be that your illness is compounded of chemical sensitivities *and* food allergies. If you eliminate only foods, you may not feel any better because of other exposures unconnected with diet – remember the 'eight nails in the shoe' syndrome? Therefore I still recommend that you follow the schedule of reintroductions as outlined in the previous few sections. You may pick up a surprising reaction from something you didn't suspect.

You must now consider the problem of chemicals. To find out more about this and how to proceed, turn to the next chapter.

SUMMARY

- Eat well before contemplating a fast. The exception is if you have had only one or two days on the exclusion diet and want to switch to a fast.
- Take vitamins and minerals for a few days beforehand; the basic formula in Appendix 6 is a suggestion.
- You may step down to a fast by having a day on grapes only (or on any other fruit of your choice). If you feel well on Day 5, you may count the grapes day as Day 1 and start testing (any food except grapes).
- Avoid outside provoking factors on a fast, such as noxious chemicals and stress; yet it is best to stay active if you possibly can.
- If you are well on the fifth day, begin testing foods. Start by introducing relatively unusual ones so as to avoid the likelihood of a reaction.
- If you do get a reaction, take a laxative and stop new tests until it clears up. You may carry on with any foods proved safe up to that point.
- If you feel no better due to the fast, your problem is unlikely to be a food allergy. Nevertheless you may be intolerant of one or more foods, and it is suggested that you follow a reintroduction schedule in order to see if you can spot any that don't agree with you.
- Go on to search for chemical allergies as given in the next chapter.

9

Chemical Allergies

As I mentioned in Chapter 2, the term 'allergy' can be a contentious one: 'intolerance' is probably a better word, certainly when it comes to chemicals. In actual fact it is sometimes hard to distinguish between hypersensitivity and straightforward poisoning. In much the same way that some adults are under five feet tall, some over six feet and the majority measure somewhere in between, so certain individuals are made ill by trace amounts of a substance, others are capable of tolerating huge amounts of it without suffering any apparent ill effects and most of us react in varying degrees somewhere between the two. It is part of natural human biological variation. If petrol fumes on the highway make an individual feel rather poorly, is that an allergy or poisoning? It certainly isn't a question I can answer; nor is it one that need concern us here. All that matters is that to remain well you must identify and remove such influences from your environment, if there are any.

This book goes into considerable detail about illnesses caused by food, but it is not really possible to consider the problem of food allergies in complete isolation from chemical reactions. My book *Your Dangerous Environment* delves deeper into this subject, but it would be inconsiderate not to give some advice here. In this chapter I will explain a little of what you need to know to sort out any difficulties with non-food substances that you may encounter; because, like food, chemicals can also cause a great deal of illness by the mechanism of hidden allergy.

Some, such as toluene diisocyanate, are deadly occupational hazards; others, like creosote or gloss paint, are harmless to most of us – yet *some* people are made ill by them. Ours is an increasingly toxic world, and if things get much worse I believe soon everyone will be feeling ill due to chemical poisons. Those who suffer at present are simply the first victims, and it would hardly be fair to consider them peculiar or to blame them for being different. It is only a question of *degree* of sensitivity.

A very gloomy book on this topic is *Silent Spring* by Rachel Carson (see Appendix 4). Its author ably covers the threat to our environment from chemicals and catalogues numerous disasters that have already occurred. Possibly the most depressing thing about the book is that it was written in the early 1960s: matters are now incomparably worse!

WHEN TO SUSPECT CHEMICAL ALLERGIES

If in the light of the self-inventory in Chapter 4 you suspect you may have allergies and yet changes of diet have not helped, chemicals may be the problem. This is especially true if several changes in diet have produced *no change whatever* in your condition. It is possible, of course, that you have no allergies at all; but if you worked carefully through the criteria of the self-inventory, this is unlikely. If you tend to get your symptoms in a particular place or *type* of location, that increases the likelihood of chemicals being to blame. Some patients are consistently made ill by entering certain department stores or supermarkets. The difficulty is that in these buildings there are large concentrations of a great variety of substances. This makes detecting one culprit rather like the proverbial hunt for a needle in a haystack.

Does your condition improve when you are away from work or home? Symptoms occurring only in the evenings or at weekends are suspiciously indicative of something in the home. Peak incidence during the day, on the other hand, might suggest an allergen at work – or even traffic fumes while commuting! These, however, are only generalisations, and there are many exceptions. Let us suppose your canteen food was poor and contained many of your allergens: you would feel unwell in the afternoons, perhaps, yet it wouldn't be the work environment that was to blame.

Similarly, feeling well on holiday needs interpreting with caution. Luckily, it is the rule rather than the exception for British allergy sufferers who go abroad. It may be the clinching proof of an environmental factor in the home or at work; on the other hand, it may be due to some change in diet brought on inadvertently. Obviously you cannot eat in France, Spain or Greece as you do in England: the very thing that is different may be your main allergen, so food cannot be ruled out so easily. If food allergies were relevant to your case, then you could have expected some clue to emerge during the diet. So, taken together with the rest of the evidence, you may feel that an improvement in your condition when you are away from home signifies a chemical problem.

YOUR SENSE OF SMELL IS A CLUE

If you have completely lost your sense of smell, especially if it was once good, this is evidence to support a chemical sensitivity. It is as if the nose becomes overwhelmed by the bombardment of substances that irritate or trigger it, and sulks. Similarly, an *acute* sense of smell may also mean allergies afoot. Very sensitive people detect much smaller amounts than the average individual because they react sooner. An extra-keen sense of smell seems often to be a prior step to losing that ability altogether.

IDENTIFICATION

The problem with chemical allergies is separating out the possible culprits: whereas most of us regularly eat only two to three dozen different foods, there are literally *hundreds* of chemicals in the average home. As soon as you step outside the front door, that number increases to thousands. Remember that quantity isn't a criterion: tiny amounts can wreak havoc. You don't have to live downwind from a plastics factory to be a victim to industrial pollution. The British Isles, green and pleasant as they once were, are now under a pall of chemical polution from our conurbations. If you travel to the far north of Scotland there is less, but it is *still present*. In fact there is a great deal of evidence that the forests of *Norway* are being damaged by the effluent gases from *our* factories. So no matter where you live, pollution is a fact of life.

Yet there is no need to despair. There is a lot you can do. It simply requires a certain amount of system in your method of approach. The table at the end of this chapter will give you some help with the possibilities, but remember, there are many others; in fact they are endless, and you may know some sources of contact yourself. Do you have a hobby or special interest? Perhaps it involves the use of some substance that could be harmful, and you were unaware of this.

Railway modelling sounds an innocuous pastime, but one patient used to suffer from severe headaches which we eventually traced to ozone from the sparks in the electric motors of his model engines. He had a layout in a converted loft which was quite badly ventilated, and the gas was able to accumulate sufficiently to make him sick – he simply hadn't realised. Fortunately, modern stock for his layout solved the problem: smoother working parts and less dirt caused less sparking and therefore less ozone. In his case, ozone has a characteristic smell which made identification easier, but this example should suffice to give you some idea of what you might be up against.

SURVEY YOUR HOME AND WORKPLACE

If you suspect chemicals may be a problem, start by making a complete investigation of your environment. Unless you are hampered by rhinitis (catarrh, runny nose), the best tool for this purpose is your own organ of smell: I call this a nose survey. I have a good rule of thumb for this, which I have not seen written elsewhere. It is this: *if you can smell it, you can be made ill by it*; meaning if there is enough of a substance to create an odour, there is certainly enough of it to cause symptoms. Go through each room in the house in turn. Imagine you are a complete stranger and ask yourself, what would he or she *smell*? Go close to objects, lift things up, kneel on the floor if you have to, and cover every surface – is there an odour from it? Polish, rubber, plastic, perfume, detergent, paint – all these smells may be present, sometimes more than one in a room.

If you can't smell anything, or you have reason to think you are so used to the smell that it isn't registering (this is normal), get a friend or a relative to help. Someone who doesn't normally inhabit the house is best, as he or she would be fresh to each perception. Don't forget to open cupboards and doors. Your clothes may not smell of dry-cleaning fluid while you wear them, but many together in the closed space of a wardrobe may give off a distinct odour. Kitchen and utility cupboards tend to act as a repository for smelly fluids such as paints and solvents; so do cellars and unfortunately these types of fumes tend to diffuse upwards and may come through the floor. What about the garage? Is it attached to the house, and if so does it bring in fumes via the kitchen access door?

THE RULES OF MASKING STILL APPLY

Remember that chemical fumes can become masked allergies, just as food can. Yet the unmasking interval varies: it is not confined to the average four days we are used to in the case of food. Really, it depends simply on how long it takes to clear from the body so that it is not protected and will react again. This period could be from four to twenty-four hours or as long as several weeks in extreme cases. Fat-soluble liquids and gases dissolve in the brain and nervous tissue, which is high in fat (this is how anaesthetics work). It can take a very long time for it to come back into the blood and be removed from the body.

Depending, therefore, on the substance and how often you encounter the allergen, it may not appear to react yet be making you ill. It is even possible to become addicted to smells. Glue-sniffing is an extreme example of this, but I have often heard patients say they like the smell of tractors or fresh paint – perhaps you know of someone. It is doubtful if the person concerned would ever connect it with allergy. Do you have a similar manifestation? If so, this is a clue. You must have this knowlege to help you if you become baffled by your investigation into chemicals. If you think you might have spotted a reaction but are doubtful, it is no use trying it again at once or sniffing it again 'just to see'. You might get confirmation, but more likely you won't because of masking. It is better to avoid that substance carefully for a few days and then try again.

There are other helpful clues. A classic give-away for chemical allergies at work or in the office is that Monday morning headache. It occurs due to the *un*masking that has taken place over the weekend. It disappears by Tuesday due to *re*masking and so remains until the following weekend, thanks to repeated exposures as you work. Look for other time-coincident symptoms like the above example and see if any of it now makes sense. You might even recognise it on a much broader scale. It is not unusual for me to be told by patients that they felt very well on their holiday abroad but that as soon as they set foot in Britain their old symptoms returned, often worse then ever. Now you see how this could be; but again, care is needed in interpretation. British food, with its many additives, could be the real reason, and not chemicals in the environment.

TESTING FOR CHEMICAL SENSITIVITIES AT HOME

Testing for chemical allergies is not very different from the procedure suggested for foods. Take the following steps:

1 Avoid the substance *strictly* beforehand. Allow four to five days to be safe.
2 Test only on a day when you are feeling well. You must have few or no symptoms for the test to have any validity.
3 Take your resting pulse before and afterwards at intervals of ten, twenty and forty minutes. A rise or fall of ten or more beats can be regarded as significant.
4 Make sure you only come into contact with one substance in the test. Give yourself a significant exposure – for example, three deep breaths – and repeat this *once* after a minute has elapsed. Take care, as this could be dangerous with some chemicals: for example, it is not recommended for poisons, such as carbon tetrachloride or ammonia.

For these and similar items it may be enough to sit a couple of feet from a dish or saucer holding about an ounce of the fluid or a bottle of it with the top removed. As the substance evaporates and diffuses towards you you will notice first the smell and then the symptoms if it is an allergen.

5 When you have tested a substance to which you reacted, you must wait until symptoms have cleared completely before trying the next one. Often this will mean no more trials for a few days.

6 As with food reactions, the bicarbonate mixture may help you to get over it. Also take vitamin C, up to ten grammes; but there is no logical reason to take Epsom salts.

Warning: Always tell someone what you are doing and have them keep an eye on you: if you pass out during one of these tests, you could be in real difficulties. Fortunately this is very rare, but it can happen.

Tell the other person that if you are overcome he or she should simply lay you horizontal, remove the offending substance and open all the doors and windows. If any has been spilt, you must be taken to a different room. *Discontinue all tests if this happens to you.* Get the help of a qualified clinical ecologist instead.

HOUSE GAS

I have used the example of allergy or intolerance to gas a number of times in this book. Perhaps you still find the idea rather far-fetched. Not so: it is one of the most widespread and insidious environmental poisons. The trouble is that its harmful effects are little appreciated, except amongst clinical ecologists; thus a great deal of human misery goes untreated because the real culprit isn't even suspected.

If you have a potty grandparent or a young wife who seems endlessly ill and unhappy, let me put in a plea on their behalf. It *may not* be a defect in their personality; house gas could be to blame. In fact this applies to a great many conditions including all the symptoms listed for you in Chapter 4. But probably the saddest group of sufferers are those who experience mental disorders such as anxiety and panic attacks, depression, delusion or depersonalisation. Rarely does anyone take them seriously; usually they are labelled as neurotic, stressed or deficient in personality. Most of them end up on tranquillisers which they can never seem to get off again. Some become frankly psychotic and spend regular periods in institutions. Yet all the time it is gas poisoning. It works just like an anaesthetic, and its effects can be just like insanity. I imagine most of you have never been in an operating theatre, but talk to any nurse who has. He or she will tell you that patients often come out with absurdities of all kinds: filth, drivel and confusion. Nobody minds because the medical staff understand that this is due to the fact that the anaesthetic gas bypasses the normal social mechanisms of the mind. (Alcoholic inebriation has the same effect.) There is nothing wrong with the person really.

Now, supposing the same thing happens in the home: the same peculiar behaviour and way of thinking, only this time no one is making allowances. The consequences can be tragic: the disruption of an otherwise calm and healthy personality; a lack of understanding from friends and relatives who thus become alienated and indifferent or even downright hostile. It's the exact opposite of what a person who is being slowly and insidiously poisoned wants: he or she needs help!

Gas causes its effects both by inhalation and also via food cooked under or over gas. This is especially true of food from the oven. Some of your food tests carried out earlier may have come unstuck without you realising that you reacted to food only because of the way it was cooked! In case you were wondering about leaks, no home supplied with gas is free of its presence: it pervades the air in minute quantities even if there are no measurable leaks. A complete seal at every joint and fitting is impossible. The amount may be so tiny that there is no smell — at least, not to the average person — but if you have read this book conscientiously so far you will be well aware that infinitesimal amounts of an allergen can make people ill. It is all a question of degree of sensitivity.

Of course, if there *is* a leak the situation is magnified many times over. Unfortunately, the gas board aren't always helpful: engineers when asked to look for an escape usually concern themselves only with those big enough to be an explosion hazard, and if they don't find one it is reported as 'No leak'! I have insisted they check a house a number of times, and each time the report was the same: nothing. But the patient had symptoms, so we were suspicious. Finally, after a number of attempts a leak was found and corrected; the patient improved. This is a recurring story.

If you think gas could be a problem in your home, get someone to check – but be very clear about what you want and why. Be pushy; sometimes that's the only way to get things done. Don't be fobbed off with a casual survey which is really nothing more than an assurance that you may strike a match indoors without blowing yourself up! If you find and eradicate a leak and your symptoms improve, so much the better. You must decide on the basis of the relative merits and problems involved whether you want to remove gas from the home and go 'all electric'. Only very rarely is this strictly necessary.

FORMALDEHYDE

No chapter on chemical allergies would be complete without mention of the worst troublemaker of all: formaldehyde (commercial name: Formalin). There is probably no chemical which is so ubiquitous in our modern world, nor one so insidious and complex in its effects. It is an ingredient of fertilisers, fungicides, insecticides, glues, laminates, certain varnishes and lacquers, medicated shampoos, germicidal soaps, mouthwashes, antiperspirants and deodorants.

The burning of organic matter causes it to be given off in variable quantities, and this would encompass bonfires, internal combustion engines, cigarette and pipe smoke, coal fires, gas fumes, the roasting of coffee beans, the toasting and browning of food, incinerators, open fires, stoves and barbecues.

Textiles are often treated with formaldehyde to improve the fastness of dyes, to make garments crease-proof, shrink-proof and waterpoof and as part of the bleaching pre-treatment of wool. Workers in the textile industry or clothing shops are particularly at risk, but you may be able to recognise the characteristic odour from your own wardrobe if you are familiar with it.

It is given off as a vapour by many plastics and polymers, especially polyvinyl chloride (PVC), foam rubber (carpet backing, furniture padding) and expanded styrene. Cavity wall insulation in the UK at present is carried out by means of expanded urea-formaldehyde foam *in situ* (UFFI), and it continues to give off formaldehyde for many years, especially when heated. In extreme cases patients have had to move home because of illness due to this noxious agent.

Food is often directly contaminated with formaldehyde where it has been used as an insecticide and fumigant, as in storage and shipping or for sterilising food containers. The tanning of leather and vulcanisation of rubber also involves the use of formaldehyde. One of my patients thought she was genuinely allergic to her husband until she discovered that it was his expensive leather coat that caused the trouble – she had given it to him as a birthday present.

Allergy to newspaper and printing inks, especially when fresh, is widely recognised, except by many of the unfortunate sufferers. Be suspicious if you sneeze when you open your daily rag: formaldehyde is the usual offending ingredient. Glossy or 'speciality' papers are worst in this respect, and new books often have a very characteristic odour. Finally (no pun!), formaldehyde is used in embalming.

Check yourself for a possible formaldehyde allergy as described above. However, you will appreciate that it is very difficult to get it properly unmasked by avoiding it. You can't, not unless you live in a very primitive society. You may need to distinguish between reactions to foods that have been treated by formaldehyde and those which have not. You may be able to tolerate quite easily a food which is uncontaminated (see Appendix 2).

SURVEY OF CHEMICAL HAZARDS

Check your home and environment against the following list of possible chemical contaminants. Any of those mentioned can and has caused severe permanent or temporary symptoms in a susceptible person. It is important that you realise that the table is *not* exhaustive – possibly several hundred more exposures occur in a single day – but these are the common important ones and should act as a general prompt. Signs of sensitivity to a chemical would, of course, include any obvious reaction that made you sick. But remember: if you find yourself liking a certain smell or it gives you a lift, be suspicious. Also, a loss of ability to smell a substance that once had an obvious odour for you is a possible sign of an allergen.

TABLE OF CHEMICAL HAZARDS

Heating
Odours from hot radiators, grilles, heating bars.
Gas fires
Oil fires
Butane/propane stoves and fires
Ducted wam air heaters
Coal fires

Cleansers (May be scented or have their own odour)
Lysol
Phenol (carbolic)
Bleaches
Soaps
Detergents
Ammonia
Polishes (for shoes, metal, etc.)
Lavatory cleaners

Cosmetics
Talc
Toilet water
Perfumes
Creams
Cleansers
Powder
Nail polish
Nail polish remover (acetone)
Aftershave
Deodorants

Fabrics
Synthetic upholstery, curtains, rugs
Printed fabrics
Clothes conditioners
Permanent pressing

Floor coverings
Waxes
Linoleum
Rubber
Foam-backed carpet
Treated (resistant) carpeting

Solvents
Newsprint
Paint strippers
Carbon tetrachloride
Chloroform
Trichloroethylene
Dry-cleaning fluid

Aerosols (fluorinated hydro-carbon propellant)
Insecticides
Deodorants
Air fresheners
Hair spray
Degreasers
Furniture polish

Medicinal
Ointments
Bandages
Impregnated dressings
Sticking plaster
Surgical spirit
Medicines
Patent 'remedies'
Rubbing alcohols
Dentifrices

Paints
Varnish
Oil paints

Polyurethane paints
Textured paint
Turpentine and substitute (white
  spirit)
Paint stripper

Motor car
Petrol
Oil
Plastic cockpit fittings
Upholstery

Leakages
Fridge
Heating boilers (flue)
Petrol/oil (garage)

Foam rubber
Pillows
Cushions
Mattresses
Lounge chairs and sofa
Carpet backing

Remember, this is only a guide. The problem of chemicals is a complex one, and for all the answers you will need to consult a clinical ecologist.

SUMMARY

● Suspect chemical allergies if you qualify according to the self-inventory but changes in diet don't seem to help.
● All the rules concerning masking and unmasking of allergies apply equally to chemicals as they do to food. The unmasking period may, however, vary and does not necessarily coincide with the four days so typical of food allergies.
● Chemicals may be the problem if you feel distinctly better (or worse) when you change your *physical location*. But you must allow for the fact that subtle changes in diet may bring about improvement as for example when you go abroad: it is impossible not to eat differently when you are in a foreign country.
● If you suspect chemicals may be a problem, survey your home and reduce exposures; then reassess. Anything you can smell has allergy potential.
● You may carry out chemical testing by challenging yourself, exactly as you did for food. Remember to allow for the unmasking period. Don't underestimate the potential hazards, and make sure someone knows what you are doing and is standing by.

- If this also fails, you must consider a number of possibilities:

1 You don't have any allergies, despite your answers to the self-inventory in Chapter 4.
2 The matter is too complex and you need to seek the professional help of a clinical ecologist. Try to make contact with one via an action group such as AAA (see Appendix 3).
3 Something else is wrong. Read Chapter 13 on hypoglycaemia and Appendix 5 on thrush. Contact your own doctor: insist upon a proper check-up or a second opinion.

Note: If dietary or chemical changes alter your condition in any way, the chances are that they are causing or contributing to it. Sorting things out may just be tough, that's all!

10

Controlling Your Allergies: How to Stay Well

Success with the Food Allergy Plan may mean that you are restored to health for the first time in many years, or possibly for the first time ever at least so far as your memory serves. This is wonderful, and it would be nice for me to take some of the credit, but really it is all due to those dedicated men and women who, despite every adversity and criticism from hostile colleagues, pressed on to discover the true facts about food and chemical allergies. It is to them that you owe your thanks.

Staying well is another proposition altogether for some. This isn't meant to be discouraging, and I would like to make it quite clear that the *overwhelming majority* of people should remain in optimum health provided all that has been set down in these pages is taken to heart and applied in life. Yet I know from experience that some of you are going to have renewed difficulties, and it would be wrong to not try to help with that situation also.

WHAT NOT TO DO

I am assuming that you carried out all the procedures correctly, felt better and continued to avoid those foods which demonstrably made you ill. If you began eating 'forbidden foods' once again because of cravings and your symptoms returned, then I think you know what to do. All you need is will-power – or common sense, whichever you are shortest on!

If your deterioration took place quite soon after reintroducing 'safe' foods, then the chances are that one or more items have slipped through the net and back into your eating pattern which shouldn't have. Return to the full elimination diet and see if that corrects it; if it does, then re-test foods slowly and more thoroughly. The rest of this chapter may not necessarily apply to you.

However, if you have been conscientious and carefully continued an eating programme which was successful at first but now seems to be leading inexorably back to illness, you must look for a reason. The likelihood is that you are developing new allergies to those foods which were safe at first. To understand how this can happen you will recall that earlier I pointed out that the frequent consumption of a food increases its 'stress' potential. The rules of adaptation will apply, and although at first your body may be quite able to tolerate this exposure it is possible that maladaptation will result from excessive use of a food. The condition is rather like a fire which by avoidance will be damped down to a mere glow but which when fuel is thrown onto it will turn into a fierce blaze. It helps us in that eliminating an allergen for a period may enable it once again to be tolerated after an interval; but it works against us when it comes to depending heavily on so-called 'safe' foods – they simply may not stay safe.

NEW ALLERGIES FOR OLD

One of the most daunting problems confronting the clinical ecologist is the patient who constantly develops new allergies: no sooner have a number of 'safe' foods been found than reactions to those also start to cause symptoms. Certain individuals trying to work out their own allergies – and you may be such a one – will also encounter this nuisance and be frustrated by it. Fortunately it isn't a very common occurrence, except among severely ill patients, but it is important to know how to deal with it when it happens.

The answer was evolved in the 1930s by Dr Herbert Rinkel, a perceptive and clever American allergist, one of the real founders of clinical ecology as a science. It is the rotary diversified diet. In principle it isn't very hard to understand. It simply requires that each individual food, instead of being eaten at random, is taken to a precise timetable. There are no 'daily' foods. Once eaten, a particular item is not then repeated for a set interval, which may be four, five or seven days. Instead it is 'rotated' with other foods, themselves eaten at fixed intervals also. To make this clearer, take beef as an example. It may be eaten on, say, Monday and then not again until the following Friday (a four-day rotation). Pork, on the other hand, may be eaten on Tuesday but then not again until Saturday, and so on.

This considerably eases the load of allergens or *potential* allergens to which the body is being subjected. If there is less exposure to any one food, there is less likelihood of it reacting. Thus this type of diet is quite therapeutic: poorly tolerated or marginal reactors may become instead very minimal and non-reacting respectively. It will also reduce the chances of new allergies developing. This could be very important to people who can find few non-allergic foods. Unfortunately, these are precisely the individuals who are likely to become quickly allergic to other substances. Theirs is a difficult problem, and a rotation diet is really quite vital.

These are two very considerable advantages, but there is also a third: a proper rotation diet is also *diagnostic*, in other words it enables one to identify reacting foods. Substances are eaten infrequently so that the masking effect will not work. The key to this is allowing the body to become clear of that food before eating it again; thus previously hidden allergies will expose themselves, or if a new reaction should somehow develop it will at least declare itself and become obvious. It will not be able to make you cryptically ill; you will know, and all you will have to do is drop it from the rotation plan, replacing it with a new food that you have found safe on testing.

CONSTRUCTING A ROTATION DIET

It isn't difficult to design a rotation diet, given certain basic rules, and patients should learn to do it for themselves; after all, no one else is in such a good position to understand his or her own likes and dislikes. True, some selections have to be made for scientific reasons, but there is always scope for culinary and gastronomic preferences. A rotation diet is essentially a personalised thing: what works well for one person may not suit another (or even keep him or her healthy).

However, one very important piece of information you need before tackling one for yourself is an understanding of *food families*. Groups of plants and animals are related chemically in such a way that the body treats them as being similar from the allergy point of view; in other words, if you react to one member of a group you are quite likely (but not absolutely certain) to react to others of the same family. It is perhaps obvious to you that cabbage, cauliflower and sprouts are related, but it may not be quite so obvious that turnips and swede are *in the same group*. Similarly, carrots, parsnips, celery and parsley belong to the same family (one of my child patients pointed out how similar the green tops are). Tobacco, potato, tomato, aubergine and pepper may seem an even less likely set, but they are in fact all in the *nightshade* family. Grains, of course, go together. Wheat seems to be the worst offender, followed by corn and the others not far behind. You have read my condemnation of this group of foods in several places in this book. Collectively, they cause more problems than any other – and they are taken collectively because they *are* a family. (Incidentally, sugar cane is also a member; these are all *grasses* of some kind.)

It is important when rotating foods to make sure that *food families* are also not encountered too frequently. To help you in this an abbreviated list of food families is provided in Appendix 1. You must refer to it when working out your scheme. In general, we allow members of the same family to be taken at an interval of two days, even when specific foods are rotated one day in four. This supposes that no other member of the same group is eaten between the two. In other words, wheat on Monday, oats on Wednesday is fine; then wheat again on Friday (or barley or rice but not oats). So you will see that knowledge of the food families is really quite essential to the construction of a proper rotation diet. It is, of course, possible to eat more than one food a day! The simplest regimen allows you to eat a given food (or food family) several times on the permitted day. To give you an idea of how this works I have constructed a simple table based on this principle:

Food	Day 1	Day 2	Day 3	Day 4
Meat	beef	pork	lamb	chicken
Fruit	pears apples	grapes	banana	orange
Vegetables	peas beans	cabbage cauliflower	celery carrot	tomato lettuce
Cereal or 'filler'	wheat	buckwheat	rice	potato
Drink	apple juice	grape juice	pineapple juice	orange juice
Miscellaneous	milk	sultanas raisins	nuts	egg

The left-hand column gives pointers to the kind of food chosen. There is a meat for each day, a vegetable, a fruit and so on. The table is read *vertically*: for example, on Day 1 you may eat beef, apple, pear, peas, beans, wheat and drink apple juice or milk. Milk is placed on the same day as beef since it comes from the same animal; similarly chicken and egg.

One or two other points are worth commenting on. Potato is not, of course a cereal, but it is a great substitute. Patients like a 'filler' food, something which satisfies. Potato does this just as well as bread or oatmeal. Potato flour is available commercially and can be used in the same way as ordinary flour, though it doesn't behave in the same manner when used for cooking.

If you were allergic to cow's milk, soya milk might be an acceptable substitute. Of course, it must only be drunk on Day 1, along with peas and beans, also members of the family of *legumes* or *pulses*. Furthermore, most soya milk preparations contain cane sugar, thus you would not be able to eat this substance on any other day.

You will see that fruit juice from the appropriate source is used to drink each day. In *addition* to this you could take a herb tea. Spring water is acceptable at any time.

AVOID DEFINITE ALLERGENS

It is important to stress that you should not include foods to which you know you are allergic. It is better to avoid these for a few months and then test them in accordance with the instructions given in Chapter 6. If at that time there is no reaction, you may then include that food in the rotation scheme, making due allowance for food families.

Eat only organic foods on a rotation diet. Manufactured items are not permitted, because of the diversity of additives. Some of these relate to food families. For example, monosodium glutamate is derived synthetically from corn. Since it is a widely used 'flavour enhancer' you would risk being exposed to this food (corn) on a number of successive days. 'Complex' foods are similarly unsuitable: a beefburger may contain not only beef but onion, wheat, corn, soya and several other items which cut right across the rotation plan. You will readily see that these kinds of foods cannot be accommodated. Thus the rule: *eat only simple unprocessed items bought fresh.*

Once you have worked out a successful rotation diet on which you feel well, it should continue to support you in good health, perhaps indefinitely, barring any adversity or stress. That means many of your formerly allergic foods can be avoided for long periods; thus you may lose many food allergies by regaining your tolerance. Eventually, you should be able to enjoy in moderation, many of your favourite indulgences. However, it must be stressed that these must only be returned to your diet on a rotation basis, otherwise you will soon be in trouble with them again. Remember: you may lose your individual allergies, but you are unlikely to lose the tendency to develop them.

EXTENDING THE ROTATION DIET

The above diet is fairly simple and can be extended in a number of ways: for example you may add a nut each day, a hot drink, a cold drink, a fish and so on. The only practical limits on this are just how much complexity you can allow without getting confused and making mistakes and how many safe foods you can find. Keep food families firmly in mind when making an addition, and don't cross these; in general, add similar foods on the same day. Nevertheless, you may find you are able to tolerate members of the same family on alternate days: to some extent this is a case of trial and error.

MORE SEVERE CASES

Unfortunately, this straightforward approach may not be enough. Some people – again, usually the severe cases – need to follow a stricter set of rules in relation to rotating in order to be successful. How do you know if this applies to you? Well, it's fairly simple: if you felt well for a week or two on the elimination diet and then your symptoms returned, and then the same thing happened with a simple rotation diet, you must place yourself in the category of those quick to develop new allergies. In effect, you are an extremely sensitive person, intolerant of foods and, by inference, of chemicals also.

Your task will be to work out a rotation diet based on the principle of 'One food, one meal'. This may sound drastically restrictive, and in fact it is; but in almost all situations it is better than feeling ill. It will keep you fairly skinny – but if you feel well again, do you really care? Besides, if you have followed the book so far and understand about food addiction you will realise that being plump or 'meaty' is far from being healthy. This is especially true of babies where round, chubby features and a ruddy glow are so much admired. It is a totally false standard of health.

No one wants you to be emaciated, but there is a happy weight for you which is doubtless lower than your friends think it should be. Don't let them worry you with ignorant concern.

I've prepared below a sample of this kind of diet. This time it is rotated through seven days. That means you must have twenty-one safe foods. If you just haven't got that many, then you will need to shorten it to maybe a five-day rotation. In this case the risk of your tolerance breaking down is proportionately higher. It would be better to include some rather exotic items to which you are unlikely to be allergic.

Spring water is permitted at any time. Moreover, you may be able to tolerate one cup of herb tea, but this must also be rotated (there are many varieties to choose from).

Example of a seven-day rotation diet for severe allergies

Meal	Day 1	Day 2	Day 3	Day 4
Breakfast	grape-fruit and juice	grapes and juice	orange and juice	oatmeal and herb tea
Lunch	cooked lentils	baked plaice	steamed broccoli	melon
Dinner	beef steak	pork chops or roast	chicken	lamb chops or liver

Meal	Day 5	Day 6	Day 7
Breakfast	pine-apple and juice	poached eggs	banana and herb tea
Lunch	baked potato	swede mash	steamed trout
Dinner	poached cod	turkey	rabbit or venison

Paste a copy of your final workable diet on the door to the refrigerator, or somewhere in the kitchen, to serve as a reminder. It is surprising how quickly you learn it by heart.

PROBLEMS WITH THE ROTATION DIET

It is possible for your tolerance of a food to break down, even on a rotation diet. This could be caused by extra stress or an acute illness, or by exposure to some other type of allergen such as a gas leak. It is unfortunate if this happens, but very important that you know how to deal with it. The key to this is forward planning. As soon as you succeed in making the rotation diet work for you — that is, as soon as your symptoms subside and stay that way — at once begin testing to identify new and useful foods. Don't wait until the problem arrives before solving it; be ready.

After a week on the diet, *all other foods are now unmasked*. You can test one or two, following the usual procedure. Any that you find safe can be held in reserve in case you need them. You don't need many, especially if you pick items from rare families that will fit more or less anywhere into the rotation without cutting across the scheme. Don't spend too much time experimenting if it makes you ill; concentrate on maintaining your well-being instead. Just do this step before you need to. If a food does start to cause a reaction, you will then be able to substitute it at once.

The following examples are foods which are to all intents and purposes separate families in their own right: eel, horsemeat, pigeon, carp, guava, brazil nut, papaya, kiwi fruit (Chinese gooseberry), sweet potato, sesame and yam. Not all of them are easily available unless you happen to live in a large cosmopolitan city, with multiracial groups and shops; but the principle is important. By consulting the more extensive list of food families given in Appendix 1 you should be able to choose items that are not related to foods that you personally were accustomed to eating.

As the weeks and months go by, you will be 'resting' quite a lot of foods and should recover your tolerance of many of these. At this stage it is worth testing and introducing some foods solely for the sake of variety. You can begin eating new substances and give old ones a rest. This way, although you may only eat twenty one foods in a week, you could be cycling through a 'repertoire' of twice that number. The only limit is how many you can keep track of without becoming confused; naturally, you should try to avoid mistakes. If it does become necessary to omit a food which was formerly safe, wait about three months and try again. If it no longer reacts, re-include it in the rotation if you wish. If it still causes symptoms, leave it for a further six months and then try again.

EXTREME CASES

The other great problem you will encounter on making this diet work for you is the question of organic foods. If you are so exquisitely sensitive that you need the diet, then it is almost certain you will be unable to cope with the chemical adulteration of food produce: vegetables are sprayed; fruits waxed or, when dried, bleached and oiled; animals force-fed on fattening chemicals and poultry treated with hormones. Then there is the problem of packaging and shipment: bananas are treated with ethylene, meats wrapped in polythene and juices put in cartons waterproofed with a corn derivative, to give just a few examples.

The problem is really quite a complex one. There do seem to be people who react to almost everything in their environment. Théron Randolph calls them 'universal reactors'. This is a distressing state to be in: it really does seem to be the case that the world they live in is too hostile to cope with. 'Total allergy syndrome' is a dramatic-sounding journalistic phrase to describe this unfortunate affliction (a term never used by ecologists), and you may read bizzare stories about it in the popular press. Ecologists find these cases reported rather regrettable: it is important that the public do not form an impression of allergy sufferers as freaks and crackpots, which is how these wretched sufferers are often portrayed. Our campaign is to educate the public to the view that allergies are not only 'normal' but quite common.

If you are among those who are made ill by so many factors that they cannot escape from enough of them in order to feel any better, it is pretty hopeless trying to go it alone. It would be far better for you to contact a professional clinical ecologist through Action Against Allergy (see Appendix 3).

11

Children as Special Patients

CHILDREN AND THEIR DIETS

Imagine being completely unable to help yourself and relying on others for your welfare. Suppose those in charge of you pumped you full of noxious foods that poisoned you (in effect) and made you feel sickly, irritable, fretful and dazed. Then they blamed *you* for misbehaving and being 'naughty' when all the time you were unable even to think straight. You tried to refuse some of these foods but were made to eat them because those who controlled you insisted mistakenly that you *must* eat them because they were 'good for you'. You would get pretty fed up with this state of affairs, wouldn't you?

Well, of course you would; yet this is the lot of many children with food allergies. A large number of children are made to eat things they would be better not to because of ignorance or myths concerning the value of certain foods. One of the common errors is that milk makes you strong. The truth is that, far from being essential, it is one of the most pernicious foods known, and many people avoid it all their lives and only feel ill if they take it. Another fallacy is that sugar provides energy: in fact, it saps it faster than any substance you can eat – it only *appears* to give energy because it creates the lethargic feeling in the first place. There are many others which I need not list here. And all the while cunning advertising sales campaigns are busy daily adding falsehoods and misinformation to the confusing pile of 'facts' that the poor, besieged housewife has to cope with in trying to feed her family well.

A child's preferences *may* be a guide to you. A strong aversion to a particular food may be nature's way of pointing out that it is an allergy, thus parents should *never* force their children to eat foods they dislike. Yet the other side of the same coin is that once food addictions have become established, then the child's 'preference' is really only a craving for an allergy food. So when it comes to the diet I usually advise parents to tell the child that he or she may *not* eat the banned foods but is not *compelled* to eat the allowed ones. This puts hunger on your side: the child either eats the right food or goes without. After a day or two of sulking and getting over the withdrawals, the child will invariably co-operate; yet he or she has the option of avoiding foods that are deeply and instinctively disliked. The difficulty I always find during this period of laying down the rules lies with the parents: to many of them it seems downright heartless to be so unyielding on the subject of what their youngster may or may not eat. I only ask them to try, and in most cases it works very well.

The fact is a lot of children are faddy eaters because of their addiction to the wrong foods. Parents sometimes complain that their child already eats very little, so further restrictions mean they may not eat at all. I explain that this faddishness is really due to the fact that the child is being poisoned by what he or she is already eating. As soon as the bowel clears of these harmful substances, the child's appetite always returns and little Johnny will often show an astonishing gusto for eating where before he showed only apathy and indifference to food. In the meantime, the previous paragraph applies. *If the child does not eat on this plan, he or she will get well nevertheless. It is vital to understand this.*

DOES YOUR CHILD HAVE ALLERGIES?

The self-inventory in Chapter 4 will provide you with many clues that may make it obvious that your child has allergies. Nevertheless, many of the symptoms are very subjective: you wouldn't know if your child were experiencing many of them. Accordingly, I have supplied below a table of objective signs and observations that may help you to decide. Once again it should be pointed out that the symptoms may have other causes, but the more of those below that are positive, the more certain it is that the problem is an allergy:

Faddy eater
Abnormal episodes of bad
   temper, tantrums,
   moodiness or crying
Persistent bed-wetting
Red or itchy eyes
Asthma
Itching skin
Rashes
Eczema
Dermatitis
Mouth ulcers
Tummy pains, flatulence,
   abdominal distress
Abdominal bloating
Constipation, diarrhoea or
   variability of bowel
   function
Catarrh, runny nose
Frequent, unexplained
   sneezing
Feeling unwell all over
Shaking in the morning
Aching joints or muscles
'Growing pains'
Headache (including
   migraine)

Irritability
Convulsions, fits, blackouts,
   'blank spells'
Frequent urination
Nausea
Vomiting
Giddiness
Excitement or sillyness
Sad
Dull
Mood swings, high to low
   and back again
Sudden tiredness after eating
Insomnia, restless at night
Always on the go, very active
Destructive, smashing up
   attacks
Eating binges
Difficulty waking up in the
   morning
Totally drained and exhausted
'Flu-like state' that isn't flu
Very pale
Dark rings under the eyes
Puffy face, swollen eyes

Children suffer from food allergies just as adults do, and some have a very hard time of it. The typical victim would be fussy with his or her food, eat poorly, have frequent coughs and colds, sleep badly and seem endlessly naughty. Skin rashes are very common. Many children end up having their tonsils and adenoids out in a desperate attempt to tackle the problem of recurring infections, and all the while unsuspected, it is something in the diet which is the cause of the trouble.

The relative frequency of allergy foods for children also seems to differ somewhat from the adult table of offenders. For grown-ups the 'top of the league' are wheat, corn, milk, egg and chemical additives; for children, these seem to be milk, colourings and chemicals, corn, then wheat (in that order).

ELIMINATION DIETING FOR CHILDREN

Youngsters may pose special problems when it comes to elimination dieting. In some ways they are better able to tolerate special diets than adults. Perhaps this is part of a child's conditioning to do as he or she is told – I don't know. Certainly many of my young patients are extraordinarily understanding about their condition. When offered something to eat which is not permitted, they will refuse politely and explain why, sometimes to the chagrin of the offending adult! We should credit them with a sensible basic nature and an intelligent desire not to be ill. Who wants to feel ill? Adults don't, so why should children?

On the other hand, the opposite is sometimes true. A youngster may have a very trying time on the elimination diet. Probably he or she does not understand the explanations given, and since he or she cannot see the reason for the restrictions, does not co-operate. These are among the most difficult cases of all, because the truth is that if children want to cheat it is always possible for them to do so. One young boy I know was accustomed to sneaking out of bed at three in the morning and emptying the sugar bowl whilst his parents slept. His mother said she had noticed the family seemed to be consuming a great deal of sugar but never tumbled to what was happening until she awoke with a headache one night, got up for an aspirin and caught the miscreant in the act.

The children who fall into this latter category actually need much more support and solicitude. It is tempting to admonish them for being 'naughty', but really it should be remembered that the withdrawal symptoms can be quite distressing and that scolding will only lower their spirits still further. It's a tough diet for an adult who is well motivated, so it is certainly tough for a child. Encouragement is what is needed – admiration, even.

It will certainly help if the grown-ups and siblings can join in on the diet. For one thing, this will give the rest of the family a vivid idea of what it takes to go through with the programme. Also – and this is quite an important point – it will help the child not to feel different or peculiar. There is one other practical reason why families should join in. From what you have read you will realise that it is most unlikely that a child with allergies is the only one in the family to have them. After all, he or she only eats what is offered; if the child's diet is faulty, then so is that of the rest of the family. The probability is that the mother or father also has the problem, perhaps without realising it. But there is only one way for parents to find out for sure, and that is to try the Food Allergy Plan for themselves. Almost everyone feels better on the elimination diet once the withdrawal phase is over, so it is worth a try.

Mothers can be difficult. There is an image of motherhood, beloved by all, in which she is a fountain of 'goodies' such as cake, sweets, buns and delicious puddings. Children, sadly, may judge her love for them purely in terms of this rather artificial archetype. It is all very well in the pages of Enid Blyton, but in real life such outpourings from the kitchen can be deadly: yes, deadly, countless husbands die early because of a wife's well-meaning ignorance in the kitchen. Thus mothers (and fathers too) may try to be 'kind' to the youngster by allowing sweets and other forbidden treats on the diet. Of course, in the long term this is hardly being kind; it is downright irresponsible and may rob the child of his or her rightful recovery. It is simply not possible to cheat 'slightly' on this programme and expect results. We are trying to *clear the bowel*, and this cannot be achieved unless the regime is adhered to strictly.

Neighbours and relatives can be obstructive for the same misguided reasons. Not understanding what it is that you are trying to do, they may feel the child is being deprived and reason that it is perfectly all right to defy your wishes in this matter. My advice is that unless you can be quite certain of co-operation you should keep the youngster away from the care of family and others for the period in question. It is only a week or two, and this should pose no strain on family relationships.

GAMES AND REWARDS

There is no doubt at all that the best way to ensure the co-operation of children is to induce them to follow the diet on the strength of their own decision to do so. One of the best ways to do this is to make it into a game. If there are rewards for eating properly, commensurate with their idea of the effort involved, it will usually be a success. There are as many ways to do this as there are children, but it is a good idea to have rewards on a day-to-day basis, since the attention span of youngsters is notoriously short. This can be followed up by a larger prize for achieving a whole week of successes. The old black marks and stars idea is good for many more miles yet. There could be stars for each successful day and a gold star for the week. Black marks would, needless to say, go unrewarded and would jeopardise the weekly score, which should be punishment enough in itself.

It should be emphasised that this is far more satisfactory than the use of force or punishment to ensure compliance, which smothers initiative; besides, the child may reason that the diet is worse than any punishment you might inflict, in which case you cannot hope to succeed! But a much more important point is that he or she will have enough to cope with that is unpleasant, at least for the first few days, without your adding to the misery. Have confidence in your child: it is amazing the number of frightful, disobedient monsters that settle down and become placid and sociable after a few days without junk food and sugar pep. You could be in for a pleasant surprise, but you will never know unless you loosen the reins a little.

It might seem silly to point it out, but perhaps it needs saying: sweets and other diet items should not form part of a reward system. Try to cultivate the point of view that they are harmful, not something kind parents give out. Thus don't be tempted into making sweets the *big* reward when it is all over – that encourages the wrong attitude. You want the child to completely change his or her thinking, permanently, not just 'until it's all over'. You see, the chances will be quite high of having to go on avoiding certain foods if the child is to remain healthy, so in that sense it will never be 'all over'. Perhaps you need to revise your own thinking on the topic, too.

SCHOOL MEALS

It is definitely easier to manage the diet of pre-school youngsters than that of older children: at home you at least have a fighting chance of controlling what they eat. School meals are particularly disastrous and must be avoided at all costs. It is sometimes possible to secure the help of a teacher in supervising what the child eats, but make sure this is someone you can depend on or you may face ridicule for your ideas and possibly open contempt of your requests. Unfortunately, there is a general misconception among teachers that because they are held liable for the safe custody of a child at school the parents' wishes don't count for a thing when it comes to the child's management.

It is undoubtedly best if you can bring your child home for meals at lunchtime. If this is impossible, the options are to provide a packed lunch within the guidelines of the elimination diet or to wait until a school holiday. Trust the school staff only if you are *sure*. The trouble with packed lunches is twofold and probably obvious to you at once. The most convenient foods, such as bread, are banned on the diet. Sandwiches are out! Moreover, even if you do send your child off with a tasty and entirely permitted lunch in a box, there is no guarantee that it will be eaten. As every child knows, 'swapping' fare is a perfectly legitimate way of livening up an otherwise boring meal. But that's the last thing you want to happen. Use this approach only if you can trust the child implicitly.

ACADEMIC PERFORMANCE

Talking about school meals and teachers makes this a good place to stress again the relationship between food allergy and academic performance. I would like to refer you once more to the case of Maxine, quoted in Chapter 4. One of the commonest of all manifestations of allergy reported is a disturbance in concentration and alertness. Dyslexia (an unproven entity) may be associated with this phenomenon, and if this were true it would be nice because it would make it very treatable. Certainly when being tested at my clinic, children sometimes react to food and other substances so strongly that they become unable to read and write or to decipher characters correctly: comprehension is lost, and images may be inverted. The trouble with calling it dyslexia, as I said earlier in connection with a 'fancy' diagnosis, is that it detracts from the real cause and implies knowledge of a condition which does not exist by the mere virtue of giving it a name. There are, moreover, cases where handwriting and word comprehension deteriorate to sheer illiterate nonsense under the effect of a bad allergen. The difficulty comes and goes according to diet, and for this reason the unfortunate child may be judged careless and inattentive at times, or even wilfully disobedient, which is most unjust in the circumstances.

Many retarded schoolchildren start to improve enormously in performance as soon as their allergy foods are identified and removed. They were retarded all right, but only by bad diets! It is vital for teachers to be in possession of this knowledge if they are to avoid meting out unnecessary and unwarranted punishment. Obviously, if a pupil were to consume a quantity of food he or she was susceptible to before a class he or she would be very likely to be rendered incapable of useful study. This is particularly true after lunch. My estimation of school dinners was never very high, but the modern offerings, with a swing towards fast foods such as sausages and burgers, are a recipe for disaster.

To me there is no more certain way to ruin the potential of a young life than to lay such extreme emphasis on academic performance as we do and yet to expect our kids to succeed while coping with some of the diets that are forced on them. That the education committees concerned serve these foods as a 'convenience' (to them) and an effort to economise is to me intolerable. Are we to sell out the future of our children, their aims and achievements, merely because town hall bureaucrats wish to cut corners in their financial planning? The trouble is that the majority of civil servants who run our lives were themselves no great shakes at school, to judge by their obvious lack of performance in cerebral functions. Perhaps they have 'tame' dieticians who tell them what they want to hear, but by all appearances they scorn advice from concerned nutritionists and listen only to accountants bleating about figures and balance sheets. But of course, even here, the deficient reasoning of the institutional mind is very evident. Cheap, inadequate meals are a completely *false* economy. Rather like 'saving money' by not servicing a road vehicle: in the end, the real cost is many times higher than doing it right in the first place.

THE FEINGOLD DIET

Hyperactivity in children is a new condition *created* by the mass technology of our oh-so-smart society: it was not diagnosed until recent decades. Partly, the reason may have been that no one knew it existed and therefore didn't look for it, but that would only account for a few overlooked cases. The fact is that it is measurably on the increase, and the reason is not hard to find: this unpleasant affliction is a direct offshoot of our deteriorating diets riddled with junk, sugar and chemicals.

There are many degrees of it, of course. Not all cases are severe and debilitating; sometimes the child seems no more than unusually naughty, restless, irritable and unable to sleep a full quota of hours. Parents often fight the diagnosis as if it were something to be ashamed of. Perhaps psychiatrists, who unfortunately usually end up treating the condition, are to blame for not recognising that it is an ecological disease not a character deformity. Some doctors, especially psychiatrists, who hate to admit any of their precious diseases have a merely physical basis, will deny any connection with diet. They would rather treat a child with tranquillisers and soporific drugs than take the trouble to work out *why* he or she is over-emotional, racing around frantically, hardly sleeping, pale and sickly, with dark rings under the eyes and self-willed to the point where sometimes it seems he or she is not even under his or her *own* control, never mind that of the fraught, exhausted parents.

Nevertheless, the dietary basis of hyperactivity has been well established by the work of many competent doctors. I myself have seen enough cases recover fully on a simple elimination programme to no longer feel the need to question this point. I believe only those practitioners who don't take the trouble to *look* will miss the connection.

One of the interesting and well-known pioneer diets in this field is that of the American paediatrician Dr Ben Feingold. He thought he noticed an association between hyperactivity and aspirin-sensitivity in children. If he were right, and aspirin or aspirin-like substances (called salicylates) made children hyperactive, then avoidance of these and similar chemicals as food additives should benefit the condition. So he tried putting these children on diets which avoided foods (mostly fruits) which contain natural salicylate substances (these include peaches, plums, raspberries, grapes, oranges, apricots, cucumber and tomato), and was gratified to observe that this produced a measurable improvement. He then went further and suggested the removal of foods containing colourings, preservatives and chemicals. This, too, seemed to be of some help.

The fact that his reasoning was incorrect – at least in my opinion – does not detract from the enormous scientific importance of his contribution to child health. But he made two significant mistakes. To begin with, diets avoiding colouring and so on must of necessity be different in other ways as well: it is a mere assumption to attribute the change to avoidance of chemicals alone. Could it not be due to the absence of *other* factors in junk food which were being omitted at the same time? Experience suggests it is. Secondly, his work did not go far enough. Chemicals *are* a problem to allergic patients, especially to children; but other foods cause much more trouble more often – milk, for instance. Corn is also a serious allergen, and yet it is a widespread ingredient of manufactured food: it is, for example, used as a sweetener in lemonade and colas. It would be true to say that where chemicals appear in food, so does corn in most cases.

So although he pointed the way his dietary modifications are too limited. Many hyperactive children simply do not improve on the Feingold diet, and that is the final condemnation. Besides, in Britain at least, few children are ill on diets rich in fruit; as a rule they are eating too many 'fast' foods high in carbohydrate when they become hyperactive. The more thorough investigations of the Food Allergy Plan are much more likely to yield beneficial results if your child is afflicted in this way.

PREGNANCY

Needless to say, a discussion on children and their allergies ought logically to include a consideration of how the diet applies to pregnant women. There is no reason to avoid the plan because of pregnancy: in fact, quite the opposite is true. It is a depressing fact that these days a great many babies are being *born* with allergies. The mother's eating habits are, unfortunately, often to blame: if she eats badly, and her diet includes many stress foods, the child may be exposed to sufficient quantities to develop reactions to these substances. By eliminating high-risk foods the mother is in effect treating two patients at the same time: herself and the foetus.

As you were told in Chapter 2, studies show that if one parent is an allergy sufferer there is a strong possibility that the child will be one also and that if both parents are so affected that risk is dramatically increased. Thus if the mother herself has known allergies, and especially if her husband has too, she would be wise to anticipate difficulties for the child and to act accordingly. This means taking precautions at the outset to minimise the foetus's exposure to allergens.

The way to do that is to follow the Food Allergy Plan; it is a low-allergy diet and so makes sense for pregnant women. There are no hazards to it. If it is carried out properly she will not be undernourished, and for many women it actually represents a great improvement in nutrition. Going without bread, cakes and sweets may seem a little harsh at first, but be quite clear: these are *not* healthy foods. They provide no vitamins and minerals but may actually interfere with the absorption of these vital substances. If you eat well from the selection of allowed foods, you will be providing your baby with the best possible nourishment.

Ignore those who say milk is essential in pregnancy. It is not true. Milk is a high-risk food and, as stated in Chapter 2, it is a very *un*natural part of our diet. Don't worry about being deficient in calcium: the idea that nature had our species born doomed to lack of calcium, salvaged only in the last few thousand years that we have been tending cattle, is patent nonsense. By all means take a calcium supplement if you wish to be sure – it won't do any harm. But remember, animals don't drink milk after infancy or take calcium tablets, yet their offspring are not born with rubber bones and teeth!

Follow the steps of the programme in the normal way. Care is needed only if the withdrawal reactions become quite severe; in that case, ease off by restoring some (not all) of your diet, waiting until things settle down. Then gradually remove the remainder of the banned foods, perhaps one every few days. It takes longer but is less drastic for either you or the foetus. The testing steps are the same, and no special precautions need be observed. However – and this is a *vital* point – just because you are not sensitive to a particular food does not mean that the baby isn't. Remember the banned foods are *likely allergens*, so it can be argued that even if you yourself don't need to eliminate those foods it would be a good idea to continue doing so for the baby's sake. Investigations show that babies born to mothers on the elimination diet have far fewer allergy problems and actually fewer health problems of any sort.

As a final word of interest on this topic, it was one of my patients who suggested the possibility that sometimes when the mother feels ill due to eating a food this might be because of the baby's allergy. It is a fact that sometimes because of her pregnancy a woman begins mysteriously reacting to food that did not trouble her previously. The idea that this could be the reason is new to me, and I haven't yet had the chance to check this out, but the possibility is certainly a most intriguing one.

ONE STEP AHEAD

For those women with time to plan, the best time to look ahead to baby's health is before you become pregnant. It is a curious fact that humans go to a great deal of effort to get animals into peak condition for breeding, and yet we don't trouble to do the same for ourselves. Farmers are very familiar with the fact the sickly, ill-fed stock breed young in similarly poor condition. Prize animals are given the best of all they require in the way of good food and nutritional supplements before going to stud. I think it is high time we started applying this principle to parents-to-be.

Mrs Belinda Barnes thought the same thing, and took the trouble to do something about it. She set up a society called the Foresight Association (see Appendix 3) which is campaigning very successfully to get this point of view across to couples intending to start families. She and FA enjoy a great deal of respect from clinical ecology doctors, and if you would like to know more about this subject or want advice at a centre near you, you should contact this association. It is self-financing, and a great deal of fund-raising effort goes towards making money that is given in support of worthwhile scientific research carried out in the field of nutrition and allergy. It is a sad fact that clinical ecology is the Cinderella of medicine when it comes to huge government handouts. This is a pity because it could relieve the National Health Service of its overwhelming burden of having to care for such large numbers of sick people. Drug companies, who normally spend a great deal of money on research, will not help because they see us as a threat. In the meantime the stalwart efforts of Mrs Barnes and her team are absolutely invaluable.

Obviously, if you are contemplating getting pregnant, *now* is the time to sort out your own personal health and get rid of those harmful foods that don't suit you; the same applies to your partner. After you have conceived may be too late. The reward of a healthy, bouncing child full of energy and free of the sadly common complaints of colic, snuffles, crying attacks, hyperactivity and the whole catalogue of 'normal' childhood problems is surely well worth the effort. You may follow up the dieting regime with nutritional supplements as given in Appendix 6. Please note that the Foresight Association has its own particular formula for vitamin and mineral tablets. This was devised in consultation with a clinical ecology doctor, so you may take them with assurance, with the proviso that *any* tablets can be allergenic.

SYMPTOMS IN THE WOMB

Interestingly, some perceptive mothers-to-be are able to recognise diet-related changes in their babies' behaviour while they are still in the womb. Sometimes there is a sharp increase in activity or, more rarely, a sudden drop. If the expectant woman realises that certain foods will lead to her being kicked within uncomfortably, she will naturally learn to avoid these substances. Probably this phenomenon is somewhat akin to hyperactivity in a child. As pointed out earlier, allergy reactions may lead either to a depression of function or to an overexcitement of it. Hyperactivity, anxiety and mania are examples of the latter. It is worth repeating that overstimulation is almost invariably followed by a reactive drop in function. Théron Randolph refers to this as 'the ups and downs of addicted life'.

NURSING MOTHERS

It is very important to breastfeed babies if at all possible as this has been shown to result in far less illness of any kind, but especially in far fewer allergies. This is so striking that one doctor friend of mine has been researching avidly for the magical ingredient of human milk that is so powerful (without any conclusive results to date, I might add). The very first liquid that enters the baby's stomach after birth appears to be crucial; if it is anything other than mother's colostrum (the thin, watery fore-milk), this seems to lead to a much higher incidence of allergies. The 'routine' hospital procedure of starting babies out with a first feed of glucose is quite wrong and can result in considerable problems later in life. Manufactured glucose is a corn derivative, one of the worst of all allergens, and can make the infant a helpless 'junk food' allergy victim before he or she is even a few days old. Cow's milk, of course, is in a similar category and hardly less troublesome than corn.

If the risk of an allergic child is very high and breastfeeding seems impractical or impossible for any reason, soya milk is a *relatively* safe alternative. There are many different brands of this product, and some are better than others. Soya milk, you will realise, is an even less natural substance than cow's milk; therefore it will hardly surprise you to learn that the incidence of allergy to soya is rapidly on the increase as it is used more and more frequently. Unfortunately, a great many allergens are able to pass through the mother's milk into the child. In this way a baby can sometimes be made allergic to cow's milk and other substances without ever having them. Don't overlook this vital fact, even if your doctor does. An unhappy baby that snuffles, cries a lot, feeds poorly, fails to thrive or has colic (any one of these symptoms or a combination) may be a victim of food allergies via the mother's milk. It is a pity that this very helpful piece of knowledge is not more widely known. Untold hours of suffering and frustration on the part of the parents, not to mention that of the baby, could be avoided by a few judicious steps if only someone knew what to do.

Believe it or not, it is possible to follow the entire plan given in this book using the elimination and challenge of foods on a breastfed child via the mother's diet. If she follows the diet outlined in Chapter 5 and the fractious, difficult or sickly infant recovers, she can then find out which foods were to blame by reintroducing them one at a time into her eating pattern exactly as if the symptoms were her own. If the return to any given food is accompanied by a deterioration in the baby's condition, that food should be avoided. Foods which cause no problems may be retained in the diet. All the rules given for behaviour of food allergies and how to test for them apply when doing this: in other words, it is no use testing the baby by having the mother eat a food which has not yet cleared from her bowel. The five-day period must elapse, otherwise the baby is receiving doses from the mother's colon, via her blood and milk, enough to keep a masked allergy in ferment.

If you are a parent, tired and worn out by sleepless nights, give it a try. I wish you luck and the baby many hours of contented rest.

Case no. 9: A child's story

Young Michael, aged eight, was addicted to candles and also to the black carbon that forms round the top of gas stoves. The former he would eat whenever he could get them, which wasn't often since his parents refused to have them in the home any longer. The latter was in plentiful supply, and no amount of vigilance on the part of his mother seemed to be of any avail in thwarting him. Sometimes he would rise in the dead of night, when even the most trusty wardens sleep, and indulge in his unique and disgusting gourmet habit.

If that was strange, it was only a beginning to the sad and complicated tale that his parents unfolded to me. Michael was without doubt mentally subnormal; yet he had not been so since birth. He had made good progress at first and now seemed to be going backwards, though nobody seemed sure why: he was now at a special school. But how bad was his condition? I listened attentively while his father explained that he was deaf; that got me interested. It is almost proverbial to me that deaf people, because they cannot hear and so often fail to understand, *appear* stupid. But when I heard that Michael suffered from recurring unpleasant infections of the ear, nose and throat, that got me *very* interested indeed. Without building up the parents' hopes too much, I suggested that his respiratory troubles might be due to an allergy. The elimination diet could help to locate these allergies, if food were the cause; then his infections might clear up, his hearing *might* improve, and then . . . well, we would see.

They agreed to start him on the plan. I met these good people several times over the subsequent weeks, and the picture gradually became clearer. Michael, it seemed, was quite a handful. Far from presenting the picture of a low IQ, he was incredibly inventive when it came to mischief: he would turn instructions completely round and do the opposite of what was required. Good with his hands, he had dismantled several objects with a screwdriver, including his own cot when he was quite young. The fact that he was really subnormal became less and less tenable as a working hypothesis, I thought. He was antisocial and uncommunicative all right, but not stupid.

Well, I'm pleased to say he improved on the diet. His tutors noticed it immediately and were soon asking questions about his treatment. For the first time it was possible to feel that communication was bridging the gap between this lonely little boy and the rest of us. He in turn responded by becoming more playful and affectionate. The exasperating wilfulness of his behaviour seemed to lessen as he became more contented and better adjusted. His mother told me with some pride that if she now asked for the door to be closed it would be closed, not swung wide — an inconsequential milestone to you and me perhaps, but not to his fraught parents. We were winning, though progress was steady and slow. We eventually established that Michael was allergic to wheat, milk, sugar and especially colourings and chemicals (tartrazine and others) commonly used in childrens' drinks such as orange squash and 'pop'. Avoiding these substances, which for him are as deadly as poisons, he continues to make good progress.

Recently he attended one of his regular follow-up visits with the paediatrician managing his case. The gentleman was rightly impressed and most interested in what we had been doing. It was then that he confided, for the first time, that Michael had been diagnosed as a case of disintegrating psychosis, a wretched and helpless collapse of the child's mind being the only considered prognosis. He admitted the mistake, which was generous of him and exciting for us; but I don't think the poor man appreciated the shock this caused the stunned parents. With such a condemning diagnosis on his records it meant that

Michael had been virtually written off. Many encounters with unsympathetic officialdom now seemed to make sense in the light of this new, sinister information. Even a dentist had one day told his mother that there was no need to explain what he was going to do 'because Michael wouldn't understand anyway'. This had astonished her because there had never been any doubt in her mind that he understood!

Luckily this ticket to oblivion has now been struck from his records, and everyone is very pleased. Michael is now simply ESN (educationally subnormal). Everyone interested in his case is watching his progress most carefully. Hardly a week passes without me hearing some new sign of his development. He is, inevitably, many years behind in learning, and it would be a fairy-tale ending to imagine that he will one day be normal, and yet. . .

The point of this story is not so much that food allergy treatment helps mental defectives; it is that eating and drinking hostile foods is a common and almost invariably undiagnosed cause for upper respiratory problems in children. Given this knowledge it should be possible to avoid many cases of 'glue ear', deafness, unnecessary illness and poor academic perform-ance due to communication breakdown in the classroom, where hearing is tricky at the best of times.

THE FUTURE

All compassionate and intelligent human beings love and care about children. They are our future: their bright-eyed inno-cence, freedom and beauty are the best we have to offer to the troubled world of tomorrow. So, really, their problems are important to us: they affect our own and the human race's survival. Unfortunately, because of our profligate waste and bad husbandry of resources, modern children are in for a tough time of it when they become adults. Our folly has bequeathed them an environment that is full of chemical toxins that pollute the earth, water and even the air we breathe on a scale never before equalled. Already this accumulation of poisons is making many people ill, and unless something is done to halt this Gadarene rush I'm sure not any man, woman or child will escape its devastating effects. For children more than adults, I hope this book succeeds. With so many years before them, sick children need all the help they can get – otherwise they may be condemned to a great deal of unnecessary illness.

12

Problem Situations You May Encounter in Elimination Dieting

EATING OUT ON THE DIET

Eating away from home will certainly be a problem on the elimination stage of your programme. Allergies still have the stigma of 'all in the mind', and even close family might not be sympathetic to what you are trying to do: expect some rebuffs. There is an unfortunate tendency in the population to view a meal such as a chop and vegetables as inadequate eating in some way; it makes many people feel uncomfortable. There is a misconception at large that a 'balanced meal', supposed to be so desirable, consists of a little bit of everything, including wheat, dairy, sugar and stimulant drinks. So if you are eating with others, expect attitudes that vary from scorn to indifference.

One thing that motivates hostility, I'm sure, is the fact that those you are with also have allergies and addictions: seeing you overcome your cravings will remind them inappropriately of theirs, since they are not able to defeat them. It is rather like giving up smoking: this seems to goad fellow smokers into every level of objectionable behaviour. Its basis is envy, plain and simple. If you have ever watched someone try to give up smoking, you may have been struck by the way 'friends' pester, wheedle and even try to trick them into starting again. Clearly, smokers like company and don't want anyone implying their habit is filthy by attempting to give it up. The same sad rules seem to apply to bad eating habits. Rather than court trouble or hostility from others whose company you keep and perhaps rely on, it is better to be discreet and keep what you are doing to yourself. Just stay at home until you have worked through the programme.

Restaurant eating is even more impractical: most menus feature little or nothing without wheat, milk or sugar, and the dieter is left out in the cold. If you can find somewhere with understanding staff that will cater to your needs, so much the better – enjoy yourself. But the usual reception, certainly in Britain, for anyone who wants to be different is being treated as a crackpot. Quite likely this will offset any pleasure you may derive from successfully eating out. Again, there often arises a need to defend the status quo, as if in saying 'I don't want your food' you are implying it is unwholesome or disgusting. Waiters and chefs are more likely to be hostile than sympathetic, but try it if you must. One surprise problem in a restaurant environment is that of odours: after unmasking a number of food allergies, it occasionally happens that food odours cause nausea. This is logical if you consider it, but hardly helpful when you are trying to enjoy your meal. Also, general food smells may stimulate urgent cravings for forbidden foods that you find really hard to resist.

On the whole it is better not to dine out during this period, but if you find you must, for business engagements or other reasons, a few simple precautions will prevent you getting into difficulties; after all, the last thing you want in front of a potential client is to be made to look foolish or a crackpot by a smart alec waiter. First of all, decide ahead of time where you want to eat. Telephone for the menu and find out if there are any à la carte items which would suit you. Licensed restaurants are usually able to serve mineral waters or juices. Choose melon (no sugar), avocado (skip the vinaigrette) or smoked salmon (this has no colouring) as starters. For the main course you can have fish or meat with salad; just avoid any sauces. It is better to avoid the dessert altogether, or ask for plain fruit.

A helpful *maître d'hôtel* can make your visit as smooth as possible in the circumstances. Just hope you don't hit on an establishment like the one a patient of mine did. A tactful phone call made in advance had appeared to have everything discreetly arranged, but in front of the assembled guests a waiter came up and said in a loud voice, so that everyone could hear, 'Ah, You're Mr So-and-so who phoned up an hour ago to ask for no wheat, milk and corn in your food'! If you find a good place to eat, stick to it. And if all this sounds rather extreme to you, do remember we are talking about a situation you would be better not to put yourself in in the first place.

Cafés are hopeless. Snacks in our modern, civilised world seem to consist entirely of tea, coffee, milk shakes, cakes, pastry, sandwiches, ice-cream and similar. These are useless to the dieter. If you must travel, stock up with a tuck bag of the things you need and take it with you. Stay away from snack bars. If you are with people who want refreshment in one of these places, have your spring water handy and ask for a glass. If you explain you are on a special diet, not many proprietors would be offended. Some patients are bold: they produce a bag of herb tea and ask for a cup of boiling water. It is easier to pull this off without embarrassment if you are with someone who makes purchases. If necessary, pay the cost of a cup of tea and ask for hot water only.

To a large extent, your own attitude dictates your success in these situations. If you can cope cheerfully through all the vicissitudes and come up smiling, the chances are that things will go your way. If you *have* to make compromises, then do so: that's only being practical, and you shouldn't feel guilty. But don't see that as a reason to abandon the programme. Fortunately, most people who have allergies will improve dramatically even with mistakes in the diet. The chances are that you are such a one, so stick with it. There is, naturally, a world of difference between being forced into a violation through no fault of your own because of circumstances and giving in because of your cravings. The chances are that you will justify the latter to yourself, thinking up perfectly 'valid' reasons why you must do so, but in your heart you will know it is wrong and that you shouldn't be doing it. Again I will stress a comment that appears often in these pages: those foods you find most difficult to give up are the ones most likely to be making you ill. When you know this to be the case, why cheat and perpetuate your suffering?

VEGETARIANS

Food allergies affect vegetarians like anyone else. The rule about allergies is that the more you eat a food, the more likely you are to develop a reaction to it, so avoiding meat may lead you from one type of unhealthy eating into another. If you felt better when you first became a vegetarian but now have symptoms, this is good presumptive evidence that you have developed new allergies to your current foods where they didn't exist at first. It is a pity some of the key foods for vegetarians happen to be stresseful, that is likely to produce intolerance. Wheat is a prime example. Moreover, lacto-vegetarians look to milk and cheese for much of their protein: these, too, are among the worst allergenic foods. Many who are committed vegetarians for humanitarian reasons eat egg since here the animal does not need to be killed; but once again this is a risky food to those with a tendency towards allergy. Those willing to eat fish have a rather better chance: at least they may ingest plenty of protein without the likelihood of problems, though there are those who cannot tolerate it, as with any food.

Strict vegans have their own difficulties, particularly in respect to animal-based vitamins (B12, for example), but less trouble with allergy *per se*. Grains are the main hazard. Moreover, it is worth pointing out that pulses (peas and beans) contain many toxins, especially if not boiled well. It would be wrong to assume they are 'safe' foods without subjecting them to the screening of this plan, especially if you tend to consume a large quantity. When it comes to the elimination diet, it is rather difficult to know what to suggest as alternatives to the excluded foods. Meat and fish are main staples of the Stone Age diet. With grains and dairy produce also banned, the list of allowed foods does tend to become somewhat abbreviated!

There are two broad approaches I suggest to vegetarians suspected of having food allergies. The first is to follow the diet more or less as given and allow themselves to eat meat, at least during the test period. For most of those who are not inclined to vegetarianism solely on religious or humane grounds this poses an acceptable temporary measure. There is an advantage here, namely that eating foods not normally eaten, even if commonplace to the rest of us, is rather like switching to exotic foods. The chance of an allergic reaction to allowed foods becomes even further reduced: certainly, if one did occur, it would be noticed at once. This approach enables the patient to avoid more of the regularly eaten foods without starving.

The second alternative is to use a fast or half-fast approach. It is drastic but will give correct answers if carried out and interpreted correctly. The half-fast would consist of one vegetable and one fruit, instead of meat; otherwise, all the information given in Chapter 8 on fasting applies in full. If you really can't face even a half-fast, follow the elimination diet with allowed food that you feel like eating. But it is very important to maintain variety: don't eat several foods over and over again, or you may make yourself ill due to *those* foods.

My experience with vegetarians is that they tend to be keen on wholefoods and alternatives anyway and adapt to new ideas rather easily. Most of them gave up eating junk food long ago. The main point of resistance, if I can call it that, is that some of them find it hard to believe that their cherished wholefoods can indeed be making them ill. But remember, I commented earlier that it is rather difficult to get *true* wholefoods these days. Whole wheat may be whole, but it is also soaked in chemical sprays added to the crop before harvesting and sometimes also in storage. If you react to wheat this might be the reason, so it will pay you to test foods correctly by my method. All the rest of the information given in this book about testing foods, organic growing, chemical allergies and vitamin/mineral supplements applies equally to vegetarians.

ALCOHOLICS

It is not widely appreciated that alcoholism is principally a food allergy problem. What the addict really craves is his or her allergy food, not alcohol; it is simply that the alcohol gives the dose more kick. The real 'fix' is with the ingredients, such as corn, wheat, sugar and yeast. This is the reason you don't hear of alcoholics who drink only wine: the alcohol content of beer may be lower, but there is nothing in wine that gives the same lift. Spirits give a bigger effect still, and many alcoholics soon progress to whisky and gin. This was easily demonstrated by giving alcoholics pure ethyl alcohol to drink: it didn't satisfy their cravings, whereas doses of the appropriately administered foodstuffs, such as wheat or corn, did.

Actually, it isn't the alcohol that causes the physical ill health of addicts, either. Cirrhosis of the liver and pneumonia are probably the two main causes of demise associated with alcoholism when it reaches dire proportions. The reason the liver is damaged is that it lacks certain essential nutrient ingredients, namely methionine and choline. These are normally supplied in the diet, but alcoholics are notorious for not eating and – despite a frequent appearance to the contrary – it is malnutrition that is their undoing. This so lowers their resistance to debility and disease that pneumonia claims a victim where these days it normally would not.

If you are an alcoholic – that is, if you can admit it to yourself and want to do something about it – use the plan. But you should also take large doses of vitamin B3 (niacin): 2,000 to 3,000 mg a day. These levels are not dangerous but may cause an unpleasant flush as a side-effect, rather like sunburn. *Eat often*: do not allow yourself to become hungry. Have a substantial breakfast consisting of fried food, such as liver, chops, kidneys and fish, with one or two extras like mushroom or tomato. Thereafter, eat something every couple of hours. It need not be a great quantity, but you must guard against low blood sugar (see Chapter 13). If you should trigger off this condition, it will bring on an irresistible craving for an alcoholic beverage. At the same time (though it is not as important at the 'drying-out' stage), take multivitamins. Those suggested in Appendix 6 are fine. This overrides instructions not to take vitamins during the plan; take lots.

Guard against stress and *fatigue* as far as possible during drying out. Your worst danger times are late afternoon and evening when you become tired.

Once you have overcome the period of withdrawal and cravings, it will be easier. Many symptoms from the self-inventory list will probably have disappeared. This should encourage you. However – and this is important – I do not recommend that you try food tests for at least a month. Try instead to continue on the elimination step for that length of time, eat well and stay well. The risk in testing foods is that you inadvertently trip a craving reaction and you are driven back to the bottle. So soon off it, you may find this too much to handle.

It is better to improve your general condition with safe eating, rest and vitamins for *as long as you can stand it*. Some people have been on the Stone Age diet for years, so it isn't impossible – it only seems that way at first!

DIABETICS

Many cases of diabetes turn out to be due to food allergies. It is even possible in some cases to conquer the disease so fully that insulin injections may be dispensed with. The dietary type, managed with hypoglycaemic drugs (such as glibenclamide), should certainly respond well. Nevertheless, it is important to take care when approaching this condition with alterations in diet. If you suddenly remove a lot of carbohydrate food from your eating (which, in effect, the elimination diet does) you could find yourself in difficulties: in other words, suffering from hypoglycaemia attacks in which you could fall unconscious. This is especially true of patients taking insulin, unless the dose is reduced in accordance with the drop in carbohydrate intake.

It is vital to let your doctor know what you are doing in advance. He or she should be able to reduce your insulin dose. If you are the type of patient who is already managing his or her own insulin levels, that makes things much easier. Even so, the condition can become very unstable for a while, and frequent visits to the family practitioner are suggested. As always, you may meet with scorn and attempts to talk you out of any self-diagnosis plan such as this diet. Don't be put off: you may even teach your doctor something!

STEROID MEDICINES

The most dangerous group of drugs in the modern doctor's armoury are arguably those classified as corticosteroids, not just because of what they may do to the patient but more because of what they take away. They suppress the body's immune reactions and may eventually undermine this important defensive mechanism so completely that the individual is left with little or no resistance to fight even the most trivial of diseases.

Nature has endowed us with a superb combative screening

system which constantly does battle on our behalf with toxins and microbes that enter via skin wounds, the mouth, lungs and other parts of the body. The white blood cells are part of this system, and their wonderful power to render harmless and ingest all manner of potential pathogens is well known to anyone who has studied elementary physiology at school. Antibodies, too, play a part by inactivating foreign matter called antigens. These are of great concern to us in the study of allergies since some allergy reactions at least are precipitated when antigens and antibodies meet. It is as if the furious tussle with the intruder upsets the furniture and makes a mess, which we call a symptom.

That is where steroid drugs come in. With certain illnesses, such as allergy reactions, arthritis, colitis and asthma, the battle is almost too much for the body and needs quietening down. Indeed, with rheumatoid arthritis and other 'collagen' diseases, the whole war seems rather pointless since, so far as we can tell, the body is attacking its own protein! Until the 1950s we were helpless to intervene in these situations; then therapeutic successes began to be observed with a (then) 'miracle drug' called ACTH. This is actually a hormone which stimulates the adrenal glands to produce their own hormones, which are basically corticosteroids. Our adrenal glands are remarkable organs lying just above the kidneys. They are endocrine, that is to say ductless, glands and secret hormones directly into the blood. The inner layer or medulla produces adrenalin. The outer layer or cortex produces a number of steroid hormones – hence the name corticosteroids. Modern drugs are usually synthetic copies of these substances, derived by chemists from the basic formula.

Steroid hormones have a number of complex actions, which are far from fully understood, including effects on sex and vitality, glucose metabolism (see Chapter 13), the distribution of fat and the density of bones. Yet their most startling property is the suppression of immune reactions. An acute inflammatory focus such as an arthritic joint settles down quite dramatically when one of these hormones is administered; similarly, asthma attacks dissipate, eczema fades and colitis becomes manageable – all this to the obvious relief of doctor and patient.

The trouble is that all this success has an important payoff:

you cannot suppress one type of reaction without doing the same to all the rest. Thus the ability to fight bacteria, which is an important and *necessary* sort of inflammation required to keep the body healthy, is concomitantly diminished. Furthermore, the adaptability of the body's systems to cope with toxic foreign substances is compromised; thus food and chemical intolerances *get worse*. Far from being a wonder drug, as they appeared at first sight, steroid hormones are actually a deadly two-edged blade that may often do more harm than good; certainly as a long-term cure they have little to offer. The trouble with steroids is the 'rebound effect' which occurs when they are discontinued. It is a very unfortunate fact that even if a disease is firmly controlled by such a medication, when the drug is stopped the complaint flares up again, *sometimes worse than ever*. In other words, there is a 'Dead if you do; dead if you don't' sting in the tail. Doctors, I'm afraid, fall into the trap all too easily in their enthusiasm to be able to offer some sort of help and, for many conditions, steroid drugs offer an attractive, if dangerous, option.

RECOGNITION

You may be unaware of the fact that you are taking a steroid-type medication. If you think this may be the case, ask your doctor and get him or her to explain. (Drug) names to look for are words including 'cort-' such as Ledercort, hydrocortisone or Efcortelan. But many are much more obscure, such as Depo-medrone. A number of well-known creams and ointments are basically steroid preparations, such as Betnovate, Dermovate and Synalar. Incidentally, do not be assured that active drugs are not absorbed from the skin when used as unguents; they are, and this is of special concern with babies, who may absorb enough in relation to their tiny body weight to constitute a *serious* overdose. Many doctors do not seem to realise this important point. Probably the best known of all steroid drugs is prednisolone. The most widely prescribed is the birth control pill, which often is not thought of as a steroid at all, yet is.

The advice you were given in connection with the drug may also give you a clue. It is important not to cease taking them suddenly. Often recommendations are given to reduce the dose steadily by one or two tablets a day. If when doing this symptoms recur, you can be fairly certain you are taking a steroid preparation.

HOW TO PROCEED

If you are taking a corticosteroid, you will want to see if you can reduce or stop this as a result of tackling your allergy problem. Extreme caution is required, but that is not to say you should not make an attempt, or several attempts, to do so. In hitting at the root cause of your illness it is perfectly logical to expect to be able to manage without any further treatment. It is important to tell your doctor what you propose to do. Only the very poorest practitioner, barely clinging onto the status of a healer, would oppose you in your wishes. A good doctor can be a great support through what may be a difficult and certainly trying time.

The essence of coming off steroids is to steadily reduce the dose. There are bound to be repercussions, and it is hopeless to expect to succeed without at least some flare-up of symptoms. Thus you should wait until the plan shows some sign of working for you before you start. On the other hand, don't wait too long because the administration of steroid drugs will cloud the issue when it comes to testing and self-diagnosing your allergies.

Be patient: you may have to try many times. There will be failures in which you are forced to return to a higher dose because of unpleasant consequences, but each time you should be able to come nearer to your objective. If there are any criteria which you can measure, so much the better; this may help by giving you a yardstick of progress. For example, an asthma patient may be able to chart the number of uses of nebulising inhaler; as the need declines, this would show on the daily record. Similarly, a colitis sufferer might measure bowel evacuations. It is surprising how, on occasion, things progress without a patient feeling any different; the objective measures will help him or her to know whether to continue in a given direction or retreat.

Finally, it may help to take nutritional supplements. I usually recommend the following:

Pantothenic acid, 500-1000 mg   Vitamin E, 200-400 IU
Vitamin B6, 100-200 mg   Magnesium, 200 mg
Vitamin C, 2-6 G   Yeast, 4-8 tablets daily

Adelle Davis, in her book *Let's Get Well* (see Appendix 4) treats in excellent detail of adrenal gland metabolism and the relevant nutrition.

SUMMARY

- Eating out on the diet is difficult and likely to compromise the stringency of the elimination. It is better to avoid doing so. Take food with you when you travel; plan ahead at a restaurant.
- Vegetarians are affected by allergies in much the same way that the rest of us are: likely foods relate to frequency of eating. The elimination stage is more restricted because of the unavailability of meat and fish for dietary use. The principles apply in exactly the same way.
- Alcoholism is basically a problem of *food allergies*, which is alcoholics' true addiction. Good nutrition is important. The avoidance of hypoglycaemia (see Chapter 13), fatigue and stress is vital to conquering this condition. Unfortunately, most have wrecked lives and suffer from too much stress to ever escape the addiction. It is all but impossible to help an alcoholic who isn't motivated to help him or herself.
- Diabetes responds very well to the food allergy approach. The elimination diet is very low on carbohydrates, and adjustments may need to be made in insulin levels in order to avoid hypoglycaemic faints.
- *Steroids*: If you are taking this type of drug, coming off it needs care. There will probably be a reactive flare-up, no matter how well you are doing on the plan. Take it by easy stages: wait until each flare-up settles down before progressing to the next increment down in dose. Vitamin and mineral supplements are vital at all stages.

13

Hypoglycaemia, the Missing Diagnosis

It would be a mistake to leave a book on food allergies without some mention of hypoglycaemia. This mimics many conditions, and can produce a catalogue of symptoms almost as complete as the one for allergy-induced disorders. The word 'hypo-glycaemia' simply means 'low blood sugar'. Glucose circulating in the bloodstream is a vital metabolic nutrient: all organs combust it with oxygen to release energy for life processes. The brain is especially susceptible to a lack of it, and the consequences if it falls too low can be as serious as a lack of oxygen. Insulin, which lowers blood glucose, was formerly given in high doses as a drug to induce convulsions in psychiatric patients, so you can see the direct relationship between brain function and glucose levels.

Because of the multiple symptomatology of hypoglycaemia it becomes difficult to differentiate from the allergy diathesis – in fact, sometimes impossible. Furthermore, both conditions may exist side by side in the same patient. Luckily the confusion is not often serious, because the elimination diet also works well as a corrective to hypoglycaemia; nevertheless, it will not cure it entirely, so it may be important for you to recognise this condition if you suffer from it.

SYMPTOMS ATTRIBUTABLE TO HYPOGLYCAEMIA

Almost any symptom can result from neurological impairment due to hypoglycaemia, though some are more common than others. Here is a list:

Sweating	Premenstrual tension
Weakness	Headache or migraine
Abnormal hunger	Frequent nightmares
Rapid heartbeat	Suicidal thoughts
Inner trembling	Tremors
Double vision	Cold sweats
Incoherent speech	Fatigue
Outbursts of temper	Exhaustion
Extreme depression	Addictions
Drowsiness	Alcoholism
Restlessness	Antisocial behaviour
Negativism	Pain in joints
Personality changes	Anxiety
Lack of co-ordination	Mania
Emotional instability	Irritability
Delinquency	Leg cramps
Nervous breakdown	Phobias
Mental confusion	Blurred vision
Light-headedness	Faintness
Insomnia	Panic attacks
Poor academic performance	

As always, it is necessary to state that hypoglycaemia is not the only cause of these symptoms. As you can see, the number of possibilities is very large, especially since most patients have several of the above in combination. There are several disorders also which may be caused by hypoglycaemia, and it is the job of a good physician to ensure that it is properly excluded as a cause in his or her routine screening tests. Among these are included schizophrenia, epilepsy, depression, migraine and asthma.

In addition to the above table there are certain other characteristic signs which point the way to hypoglycaemia. The most significant of these are a sudden attack of tiredness and hunger about mid-morning and a profound fatigue or even faintness coming on late in the afternoon. Both are rapidly relieved by eating, especially by eating something sweet. You will recognise the former as the 'eleven o'clock gap' promoted by chocolate bar manufacturers. The 'run down' feeling is due to a lack of blood sugar, so naturally any sort of candy or sweet food will relieve it immediately. The advertisers play heavily on this theme, but, as you will read below, their products are in fact responsible for causing the attack in the first place. (What could be better for profits than to have a nation hooked on sweet food, making itself ill and then only feeling better by consuming *more* of your product?) Further clues to look for are waking hungry in the night, the need to eat frequently, sometimes a panic – almost a desperation – to get food, irritability and a lack of concentration helped by eating carbohydrate foods and craving for sweet things.

A good clinician can usually diagnose hypoglycaemia from an inspection of the patient's diet. If it shows repeated eating of sugary foods, white flour, drinks with sweeteners, chocolates, sweets and perhaps alcohol, the presence of this is very probable. This sort of eating shows an addictive craving for sugar; but even if that were not the case, the over consumption of such foods would very rapidly *cause* a disorder of the sugar metabolism leading eventually to hypoglycaemia.

CAUSE

The key to this condition, as with allergies, is what the person eats. The consumption of too much carbohydrate food, ironically, causes hypoglycaemia. The exact progress of events is as follows:

1 Consumption of excess sugary food.
2 This raises the blood sugar level too fast. The body responds by releasing insulin and other glucose-regulating hormones from the adrenal gland.
3 This lowers blood sugar, but usually too fast. There is an overcompensation and the level falls too low.
4 This sets up symptoms, including hunger. There is a craving for more sweet food, soon after the previous meal.

5 The new intake sets off the above cycle all over again.
   Blood sugar levels roller-coaster up and down many times a
   day.
6 Eventually the body's ability to cope with these continuous
   rushes of sugar become exhausted. The adrenal (stress)
   gland cannot cope with the demand for glycogen-to-glucose
   conversion mediated via its hormones, and so the regulation
   mechanism breaks down completely.
7 The only thing which remains to maintain blood sugar is to
   keep eating carbohydrate food: it's a trap!

A more contentious point, but one I believe to be true, is that
this condition is pre-diabetic. After many years, possibly
decades, of this sort of abuse the insulin-release mechanism
fails completely. The pancreas gland becomes exhausted and is
no longer capable of producing this essential hormone.
Hypoglycaemia is the warning sign that trouble is just around
the corner.

From the above you will see that sugar is actually the *cause*
of hypoglycaemia. Sweet foods only *seem* to give you energy:
they appear to do so simply because they took away your pep
in the first place. The worst possible treatment for this
condition is sugar, and yet most doctors, through ignorance of
the facts, advocate sugary food and sweets to provide a pick-
me-up.

Typical hypoglycaemia sufferers eat a poor breakfast, such as
coffee and toast, or none at all. By mid-morning they need a
snack – usually cake, biscuits or sweetened drinks – and this
triggers hypoglycaemia in a matter of ten to sixty minutes. The
demand is set up for more food, and this continues all day. The
diet as a whole is often nutritionally inadequate, lacking in
protein foods, especially fats and essential oils. Eating between
meals is usual and compulsive, due to cravings. Allergy patients
will recognise the strong resemblance between this condition
and cravings due to addiction.

DIAGNOSIS

Any doctor should be able to diagnose this condition purely on
the basis of the patient's history: it is glaringly obvious to those

who know what to look for. It is also possible to make a 'therapeutic' diagnosis, that is to treat the condition as if it existed and then if that cures it to assume you were right in the first place. (Scientific colleagues cringe at this sort of approach, but what we are describing here is far safer than administering drugs on a trial-and-error basis, which is the method generally employed.)

THE SIX-HOUR GLUCOSE TOLERANCE TEST

The chief laboratory back-up is the glucose tolerance test (GTT). The patient fasts overnight, and a blood sample is taken to measure the blood sugar level at this point. Then the patient is asked to drink a concentrated solution of glucose containing fifty to a hundred grams according to body weight. Repeat blood samples are taken every half-hour, and in each case the blood glucose concentration is measured. In hospital, a period of two-and-a-half hours is allowed in which time it is usually possible to detect a diabetic response, but this is not long enough when hypoglycaemia is suspected; consequently the diagnosis is often missed, even when a GTT is done. It is better to continue the test for six hours because often the characteristic reaction takes place long after the two-and-a-half hour mark.

The results of a GTT are usually represented graphically, and three typical responses are shown below:

A normal response

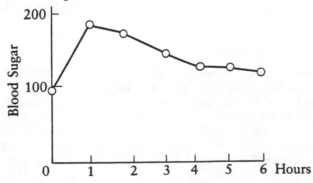

Note that the blood glucose started with a sharp rise to over 50 per cent of the starting value within one hour. Then it fell steadily, but at no stage did it fall below the fasting level, which is taken as the baseline.

A diabetic curve

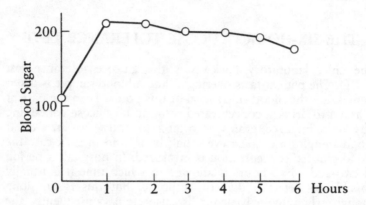

This is included for interest only. The characteristic of a diabetic curve is that it goes high and stays high, falling only very sluggishly, for the reason that the body has lost the ability to deal with carbohydrate, which is not removed easily from the blood. The test is built around a fast: apart from the test dose the patient had nothing by mouth for almost twenty hours. You will readily see that regular eating will result in a permanently high blood sugar level, which is what diabetes is in essence.

A hypoglycaemia curve

The points to notice about the following example, which came from a fourteen-year old epileptic girl, are as follows. The graph rose as it should during the first hour and appeared to be normal until the third hour, when it suddenly fell very steeply. Within an hour it had dropped by over seventy units; moreover, from then onwards it remained *below the fasting level* for a considerable time before returning to 'baseline'.

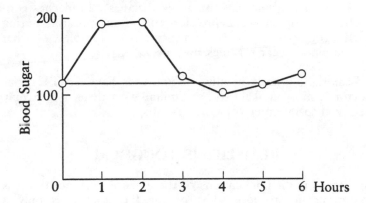

There are several possible responses which would suggest hypoglycaemia, either actual or latent. Dr Patrick Kingsley, an experienced clinical ecologist practising in Leicestershire, suggests the following criteria for diagnosing hypoglycaemia.

DIAGNOSIS OF HYPOGLYCAEMIA FROM GTT RESULTS

Hypoglycaemia is indicated:

1 When the blood sugar, in the course of a six-hour glucose tolerance test, fails to rise more than 50 per cent above the fasting level (this is rarely encountered);
2 By a glucose curve which falls during a six-hour test to 20 per cent below the fasting level;
3 By a glucose test in which the blood sugar falls fifty milligrams per cent or more during any one hour of the test (usually follows a rapid rise of fifty milligrams per cent in the first thirty minutes);
4 By a glucose tolerance test in which the absolute blood sugar level falls in the range of fifty milligrams per cent or lower (anything below sixty-five milligrams per cent is suspicious);

5 By clinical symptoms, such as dizziness, headache, confusion, palpitations, depression and so on appearing during
the course of a glucose tolerance test – regardless of what
the blood sugar readings may be.

Bear these criteria in mind if you ever have a GTT. Your
doctor is most unlikely to be familiar with them, and it may
help you to interpret your own results.

REAL LIFE IS TOUGHER!

In discussing the implications of the glucose tolerance test it is
important not to lose sight of the fact that it is only a
laboratory test: the patient is sitting comfortably and relaxed
for hours, isolated from everyday life and, usually, without any
trying circumstances to cope with. Everyday living brings a
great deal of stress that could exacerbate a hypoglycaemia
attack. What might be trivial in the laboratory could become a
major problem at work, where the individual may be
constantly under pressure, with little time for proper eating and
often access to only the wrong kind of foods. It is important to
consider the results of any test in this light. A borderline or
suspicious result is very good working evidence of a hypoglycaemia tendency in a crisis situation.

STRESS

With allergies, and indeed any illness, stress is a major
contributory factor. The body has a complex mechanism for
coping with stressful situations which, providing it is working
well, is very effective. However, if you recall Hans Selye's
theory of general adaptation (see Chapter 2) you will realise
there is a premium on this mechanism: if pressed into action
over and over again, it eventually fails. From being adapted to
the stress (Stage 2) the body defences then become exhausted
and adaptation fails (Stage 3). This applies to the constant
loading of the system with carbohydrate foods demanding to be
absorbed safely into the system.
Once again, the brunt seems to fall on the adrenal glands,

which are our principal 'stress organs'; thus hypoadrenalism is an integral part of deficient carbohydrate metabolism. If these glands are unable to respond adequately, insufficient hormone is released to order the conversion of glycogen to glucose and the blood level cannot be maintained. For that reason, and until our understanding of this condition improves, I usually advocate adrenal gland extract as a supplement along with other corrective measures. You will not be able to self-administer this substance in quantities that are useful, but at least commercially available preparations are harmless if you want to try them together with other recommendations.

PUTTING IT RIGHT

Just as diet causes hypoglycaemia, so it may cure it. A change of eating habits is the most fundamental step to recovery from this blighting condition. You must stop ingesting all refined carbohydrate forthwith. This means sugar, white flour and corn sweeteners (as used in cordials, squashes, colas, doughnuts and so on). I call these 'fast carbo' because they are digested and gush into the system so quickly that the body has no time to adapt and a rapid rise in blood glucose is inevitable. These are *stress foods* in just the same way that allergens are, and with all the same liabilities. Honey, fruit sugar (fructose) and untreated raw sugar are much gentler on the system, but for the time being avoid them also.

It is wise, at first, to limit your carbohydrate intake to between sixty and eighty grams per day depending on your size; a child should be able to manage with fifty grams. The simplest way of working out your intake is to buy one of the excellent little books on the market with the title *Carbohydrate Counter* (see Appendix 4) or similar. There you will find listed all the common foods and a guide as to the average carbohydrate content. Adding up grams from several different sources may seem rather laborious at first, but you will soon get into the swing of things and know even without looking up the figures that you are allowed a certain combination of foods. Also, very many foods are rated as nil carbohydrate content, so you can eat as much of these as you like without affecting the daily score: for example, any meats, cheese, most vegetables, fish, and so on.

Some foods you will learn to avoid altogether because they are so high in carbohydrate that you cannot eat them within the constraints of a fifty-gram limit. These are dessert mixes, cake, sweets, biscuits, breads and doughs, pastry and pasta, any alcoholic drink, certain fruits such as figs, grapes and bananas, rice, potatoes and some beans. In addition, you will have to monitor carefully your intake of a great many other foods which *do* contain carbohydrate and will therefore contribute to your daily total.

BREAKFAST LIKE A KING!

There is no doubt that breakfast is the key meal in steering yourself away from the rocks of hypoglycaemia. The average British morning intake – cornflakes, toast and marmalade, plus tea or coffee (often also sweetened) – is a recipe for disaster. It will rocket your blood sugar and trigger the compensatory plunge by mid-morning, which starts you snacking between meals. Conversely, a good breakfast will set you up with a steady rise in blood sugar, which sustains itself at a safe level for many hours to come, avoiding hunger and any triggering climbs or falls in level. By a good breakfast, by the way, I mean a *meal* such as chops, liver, kidneys, egg or fish, perhaps accompanied by tomatoes and mushrooms, with fruit to follow. Oatmeal is allowed, also whole cereal muesli, but only within the stipulated carbohydrate levels. The fatty part of the meal *should not be omitted*. There is a very good reason for this, which is that fat slows down digestion and causes a slow release of digested products from the intestine; thus there are no embarrassing rushes in glucose to the blood. Naturally, you will only breakfast on foods which are safe in allergy terms, but that will still leave you plenty of scope for a good, sound meal.

A lot of patients complain they are unable to face a large meal in the morning. I have, on occasion, told a person to eat one anyway, even if it makes him or her heave. Sometimes after ten consecutive days of vomiting after breakfast he or she learns to tolerate it and then starts making progress with symptoms. The usual problem with breakfast appetite is actually the evening meal. It is a common habit to consume a large meal after 6 p.m., which is never properly metabolised because the person then sits in front of the television and does very little physical work. Consequently on waking there is no feeling of hunger and no desire for breakfast, so that person goes to work on an empty or ill-fed stomach. This is a completely retrograde step, of course. Someone said it beautifully by the epithet we should 'Breakfast like a king, lunch like a prince and supper like a pauper.' For more information of this topic I cannot do better than to refer you to *Let's Eat Right to Keep Fit* by Adelle Davis, Chapter 2 of which is entitled 'Breakfast Gets the Day's Work Done'.

SUPPLEMENTS

Certain dietary additions will help to combat the effects of hypoglycaemia. I usually advocate the following:

Vitamin B6	200 mg
Pantothenic Acid	1,000 mg
Vitamin C	2 g
Niacin (vitamin B3)	1,000 to 2,000 mg
Manganese	5 mg
Chromium	400 mcg
Potassium	1,000-12,000 mg (1 month only)

These are daily doses, divided however you like. With some of the supplements, the niacin for example, you may need to start with a smaller dose and gradually build up the amount according to your tolerance. Potassium is included because the profound tiredness and lethargy often experienced by hypo-adrenal patients is usually due to low blood levels of this vital element. Because deficiencies never occur singly it is a good idea to also adopt the use of the basic vitamin formula given in Appendix 6.

YOU *CAN* EAT BETWEEN MEALS!

This may be one of the few occasions when a qualified doctor tells you it can help to eat between meals, so pay attention! The fact is that hypoglycaemia sufferers are in serious trouble at the point when their condition becomes so manifest as to be a diagnosable clinical entity. This means that carbohydrate regulation is impaired, if not absent, and blood sugar levels may be dependent solely on what the patient eats. Because it is a long-term effect it may mean that the proper control mechanisms have been so damaged as to be irretrievably lost. More research needs to be done in this area in order for any firm conclusions to be drawn.

In the meantime, it helps greatly to space meals at regular intervals. Avoid going too long without some form of dietary intake. This is not intended to condone eating carbohydrate snacks and sweets between meals: you must confine your eating to foods that are low or completely lacking in carbohydrate. Cheese, vegetables or slices of meat will fit the bill nicely. Using small amounts of similar foods, break up your eating routine into six or eight *smaller* meals. As you begin to feel better and your attacks come under control, you may then gradually work back towards a more normal eating schedule. Even so, you must not let yourself go for long periods without food. This is especially true if you are under stress. Keep permitted foods with you on long journeys.

RECOVERY TAKES TIME

More so than with allergies, it takes a great deal of time to correct hypoglycaemia and hypodrenalism. The five-day 'clear out' lapse as used in the case of allergies is irrelevant here; in fact, it may take several weeks before you begin to feel very much improved. It is important that you remember this and don't abandon the programme too early.

It is *vital* to stop smoking and to avoid stimulants with caffeine, such as coffee. These may trigger hypoglycaemia attacks. Again, this has nothing to do with allergies *per se*.

You will probably notice a striking similarity between the hypoglycaemia diet and the elimination step of the plan. This is no coincidence: as I said earlier, allergy and hypoglycaemia are so closely bound up as to be almost inextricable from each other. Most of the toxic, stressful or maladapted foods are also carbohydrate-rich. *Nothing in this chapter is intended to get you to eat foods to which you are allergic*!

SUMMARY

Hypoglycaemia mimics many other conditions, including allergic reactions. Often the two problems coincide in the same patient. It is important to distinguish between them because the remedies are different.

● Hypoglycaemia is brought about by the intake of excessive amounts of carbohydrate, especially sugary foods, over a long period.

● Apart from symptomatic effects, the principal characteristics of this diathesis are bouts of hunger, irritability and fatigue, apparently relieved by eating sweet foods.

● Treatment is by dietary correction first and foremost. The carbohydrate level needs to be restricted to fifty to eighty grams daily, depending on one's age and size.

● A substantial breakfast, including fatty foods which are digested slowly, is the key to slow release of sugar and starch digestion products from the alimentary tract. This prevents too rapid a build-up of blood sugar.

● The victim should eat a little and often, but not carbohydrate in response to a craving. Protein foods should be the only foods eaten between meals. It is important to avoid stress, fatigue and over-long periods without sustenance.

● Certain vitamin and mineral supplements help, notably vitamins B6, B3, C, manganese, chromium, potassium and pantothenic acid. Adrenal gland extract is also recommended where under the guidance of a physician.

● Hypoglycaemia may be pre-diabetic, is a lifelong tendency, and is connected with poor response to stress. General immunity may be low as a result, thus there may be a predisposition to many other illnesses.

● It is important that, without becoming introverted to the point of neurosis, sufferers of this condition care for themselves and their diet. A stressful lifestyle and a return to poor eating will soon result in ill health, perhaps with serious consequences.

Appendices

1 Table of Food Families

The following table gives common foods and their families. No attempt is made here to list all foods or to include all biological families.

PLANT FAMILIES

Fungi or moulds: Baker's yeast (hence breads and doughs, etc.), Brewer's yeast (hence alcoholic beverages), mushroom, truffle, chanterelle, cheese, vinegar (hence pickles and sauces).

Grasses: Wheat, corn, barley, oats, millet, cane sugar, bamboo shoots, rice, rye. (Note that buckwheat is *not* a member of the grass family.)

Lily: Onion, asparagus, chives, leek, garlic, sarsaparilla, shallot.

Mustard: Broccoli, cabbage, cauliflower, Brussels sprouts, horse-radish, kohlrabi, radish, swede, turnip, watercress, mustard and cress.

Rose: Apple, pear, quince, almond, apricot, cherry, peach, plum, sloe, blackberry, loganberry, raspberry, strawberry.

Pulses or Legumes: Pea, chick pea, soy bean (hence TVP), lentils, liquorice, peanut, kidney bean, string bean, haricot bean, mung bean, alfalfa.

Citrus: Orange, lemon, grapefruit, tangerine, clementine, ugly, satsuma, lime.

Cashew: Cashew nut, mango, pistachio (also poison ivy).

Grape: Wine, champagne, brandy, sherry, raisin, currant, sultana, cream of tartar.

Parsley: Carrot, parsley, dill, celery, fennel, parsnip, aniseed.

Nightshade: Potato, tomato, tobacco, aubergine, pepper (chilli, paprika).

Gourd: Honeydew melon, watermelon, cucumber, squashes, cantaloup, gherkin, courgette, pumpkin.

Composite: Lettuce, chicory, sunflower, safflower, burdock, dandelion, camomile, artichoke, pyrethrum.

Mint: Mint, basil, marjoram, oregano, sage, rosemary, thyme.

Palm: Coconut, date, sago.

Walnut: Walnut, pecan.

Goosefoot: Spinach, chard, sugar beet.

Sterculia: Chocolate (cacao bean), cocoa, cola nut.

The following commonly eaten plants have no *commonly* eaten relatives: juniper, pineapple, yam, banana, vanilla (often a chemical imitation), black pepper, hazelnut, chestnut, fig, avocado, maple, lychee, kiwi fruit, tea, coffee, papaya, brazil nut, ginseng, olive, sweet potato, sesame (also as tahini).

ANIMAL FOOD FAMILIES

Bovines: Cattle (beef), milk and dairy products, mutton, lamb, goat.

Poultry: Chicken, eggs, pheasant, quail (*not* turkey).

Duck: Duck, goose.

Swine: Pork, bacon, lard (dripping), ham, sausage, pork scratchings.

Flatfish: Dab, flounder, halibut, turbot, sole, plaice.

Salmon: Salmon, trout.

Mackerel: Tuna, bonito, tuny, mackerel, skipjack.

Codfish: Haddock, cod, ling (saith), coley, hake.

Herring: Pilchard, sardine, herring, rollmop.

Molluscs: Snail, abalone, squid, clam, mussel, oyster, scallop.

Crustaceans: Lobster, prawn, shrimp, crab, crayfish.

The following commonly eaten animals and fishes have no *commonly* eaten relatives: anchovy, sturgeon (caviar), whitefish, turkey, rabbit, deer (venison).

2 *Organic foods*

It is impossible to deal effectively with the subject of organic foods in a book of this size. Nevertheless I have alluded to them several times in the course of the text, and a little more information may be helpful, if only to let you know what you are up against! The problem so far as the allergy sufferer is concerned is that he or she may be able to eat a specific food quite safely, without experiencing any reaction; yet because that food is not readily available without contamination it remains unavailable for general use. This can also be very misleading during tests: if a food does seem to react during testing but came from a normal commercial source, it may be worth trying to obtain a special sample, free of all chemicals, and re-testing it.

There are a number of ways that toxic substances can be present in or on your food, and it is worth listing them for clarification:

1 **By accident:** Sprays intended for a different crop may have fallen onto the one you are eating.

2 **Deliberately by the farmer:** This may be part of a husbandry programme for crops. Thus grain crops are over-sprayed many times before harvesting with powerful chemicals such as weed-killers, pesticides and fungicides. Any one of these might cause an apparent 'wheat allergy'.

   It applies also to animal foodstuffs. Chickens reared on a mass commercial scale are a hazard because of the high level of hormones and bactericides they contain. In one community where chicken was the staple, little girls of five were seen to develop breasts due to the meat's high hormone content.

3 **Veterinary reasons:** Sometimes an animal on our food chain

receives chemical treatment for reasons other than a mere desire to increase profits. A sick animal needs medicines, and the drugs given to it may appear in the meat or milk you consume. Penicillin levels in cow's milk are strictly controlled, but nothing else is!

4 **Storage:** Many foods are treated chemically to improve their storage potential. Potatoes are sprayed with tecnazine to prevent them sprouting. Wheat may receive *yet another* chemical spray, for the same reason.

I have learned that at certain ports in the United Kingdom landed fish are commonly sprayed with antibiotics. This stops it rotting so quickly and enables stale fish to reach your larder without going high. Whatever you think of this odious practice, it is clearly a hazard to those allergic to antibiotics – a common problem. I understand, incidentally, that to date this does not apply to Scottish fishing ports.

5 **Manufacturing processes:** Processed foods are notorious for the number of chemicals they contain; there are over 3,500 such additive substances, and over 1,100 are listed for legal use in Britain.

A great deal of specious argument exists on this topic. I heard one food industry spokeswoman say that if preservatives were not used foods would not last and would therefore not be consumed. My answer to that is that I would be very happy if such commodities were not in fact eaten. The problem would be at an end if we stopped buying these foods; no manufacturer could then go on producing them. This is largely a matter of education, and with big business controlling the purse-strings it is small wonder that little money is spent on this important area of health teaching.

GROW YOUR OWN

There is no doubt that the best way to solve the supply problem is to grow your own if at all possible. To make this work you don't need much land – just know-how – and it can be learned. Percy Thrower, the famous TV gardening personality, is reputedly able to grow all the fruit and vegetables for a family of four in a plot no bigger than twenty by thirty feet. For more advice on organic vegetable growing, contact the Henry Doubleday Research Organization (see Appendix 3). Also, many excellent books exist on this topic which should be available through your local library.

If all this sounds like too much trouble, don't despair: you may have friendly neighbours with green fingers who will be only too pleased to help if you explain your problem. Many amateur gardeners grow far too much for their needs at any one time, and they will be glad to get rid of any excess in a good cause. Fill your freezer. You will be able to buy produce much more cheaply this way and your neighbour can recoup some of his or her expenses. Most wouldn't charge you anything for a few organic fruits and vegetables scrounged in order to perform food tests. Just make sure they understand your requirements, however, as many keen gardeners use chemicals.

The Organic Farmers' Association (see Appendix 3) should be able to put you in touch with a farmer not too far away who can supply some of your needs. It also pays to visit the country at weekends. There are many small landholders who utilise unsophisticated techniques to rear and to grow produce. A quiet word explaining your needs is enough for most of them to become very interested in your problem and most helpful with supplies.

A useful booklet on the subject is *The Organic Food Guide* (see Appendix 4). Remember: those merchants listed are only a fraction of the ones available. Beware of health food shops in general, many of which don't seem to know what they are selling, but if you know a good one its proprietor may be able to put you in touch with a suitable supplier. A *really* good shop will actually have the produce in stock, but that is only being professional.

Also recommended is the booklet *Look at the Label*, which deals with the subject of new UK regulations on the labelling of foodstuffs. This is available from the address below:

Ministry of Agriculture and Fisheries
Publications Unit
Lion House
Willowburn Trading Estate
Alnwick
Northumberland
NE66 PF

3 Some Useful Addresses

The following are addresses you may find useful:

Community Nutrition Institute
2001 S Street, N.W.
Washington, DC 20009   (202) 462-4700
Citizen advocates specializing in food quality, food labeling, and nutrition issues. Sponsors workshops. Publishes booklets.

Cooking for Survival Consciousness
Box 26762
Elkins Park, PA 19117   (215) 635-1022
Educational and scientific foundation; disseminates information about food and cooking based on health-through-nutrition. Areas of concern include: preventive health care through nutrition, the study of diet-linked diseases, ecological and conservation aspects of food leading to alternative systems of nourishment and cooking. Publishes journal and a cookbook.

American Allergy Association
P.O. Box 7273
Menlo Park, CA 94026   (415) 322-1663
Disseminates information on diet, environmental control, and other facets of allergy advice. Publishes a newsletter and pamphlets.

Asthma and Allergy Foundation of America
1302 18th Street, N.W., Suite 303
Washington, DC 20036   (202) 293-2950
Works to solve the health problems posed by allergies. Provides information to the public. Helps develop programs for treatment and prevention of allergic diseases. Publishes newspaper and pamphlets.

Human Ecology Foundation
R.R. 1
Goodwood, Ontario
CANADA LOC 1AO

Allergy Foundation of Canada
P.O. Box 1904
Sakatoon, Saskatchewan
CANADA S7K 3S5   (386) 664-4618

Henry Doubleday Research Organization
Convent Lane, Bocking
Braintree, Essex, ENGLAND
An international charity aimed at research into organic food-growing methods. Members receive the newsletter. Advice available that is applicable to growing chemical-free foods in your own garden. Much current research into growth methods on their own farm site.

Natural Food Associates
P.O. Box 210
Atlanta, TX 75551   (214) 796-3612
Professionals and consumers interested in organic farming, natural foods, and human health. Objectives are: to expose the dangers of chemical contamination of food, water, and land and to offer preventive measures to metabolic disease. Offers books and publishes monthly *Natural Food and Farming Magazine,* monthly newspaper, and book catalogue.

Natural Organic Farmer's Association
P.O. Box 335
Antrim, NH 03440   (603) 588-2760
Promotes organic growing methods. Disseminates information and publishes *Natural Farmer.*

New England Foundation for Allergic & Environmental Diseases
3 Brush Street
Norwalk, CT 06850   (203) 838-4706
May be able to refer you to an organization in your area.

Allergy Information Association
25 Poynter Dr., Room 7
Weston, Ontario
CANADA M9R 1K8   (416) 244-9312
Publishes a quarterly publication *Allergy Shot.*

American Academy of Environmental Medicine
P.O. Box 16106
Denver, CO 80216

Price-Pottenger Nutrition Foundation
P.O. Box 2614
La Mesa, CA 92041
Purpose: to disseminate nutritional information through books, films, teaching aids, exhibits, quarterly publications and reprints of continuing research. Also involved in experimental farm projects, efforts to formulate ways of incorporating sound nutritional principles into the world's agricultural practices.

American Celiac Society
45 Gifford Avenue
Jersey City, NJ 07304   (201) 432-1207
Provides information on how to follow a gluten-free diet. Publishes newsletter.

Clinical Ecology Publications
109 West Olive
Fort Collins, CO 80524
Publishes *Clinical Ecology--Archives for Human Ecology & Disease.*

Or

Contact your local library for resources/clinics/organizations in your area.

4   *References and Recommended Books*

This is not an attempt to produce a comprehensive reading list but rather a means of introducing you to the horizons of medicine. Most of the books listed contain extensive bibliographies and reference sections which will lead you to further reading.

GENERAL

Coping with Your Allergies by Natalia Golos and Frances Golos Golbitz (Simon & Schuster)
Not All in the Mind by Dr Richard Mackarness (Pan)
Chemical Victims by Dr Richard Mackarness (Pan)
The Pulse Test by Dr Arthur Coca (Arco)
Allergies, Your Hidden Enemy by Théron Randolph (Turnstone, 1982)
Against the Unsuspected Enemy by Amelia Nathan-Hill (New Horizon)
How to Control Your Allergies by Robert Forman (Larchmont)

Dr Mandell's 5-day Allergy Relief System by Marshall Mandell and Lynn Waller Scanlon (Thomas Y. Crowell)
The Allergy Problem by Vicky Rippere (Thorsons)
Your Dangerous Environment by Dr Keith Mumby
E for Additives by Maurice Hanssen (Thorsons 1984)

CHILDREN

Tracking Down Hidden Food Allergies by Dr William Crook (Professional Books)
Allergies and the Hyperactive Child by Dr Doris Rapp (Sovereign)
Food for Thought by Maureen Minchin (Alma)
Are You Allergic? by Dr William Crook (Professional)

FOR DOCTORS

Food Allergy by Herbert Rinkel, Théron Randolph and Michael Zeller (Charles C. Thomas)
Brain Allergies, The Psycho-nutrient Connection by Dr William Philpott and Dwight K. Kalita (Keats)
Human Ecology and Susceptibility to the Chemical Environment by Dr Théron Randolph (Charles C. Thomas)
Clinical Allergy by Dr Harris Hosen (Exposition Press)
A Physician's Handbook on Orthomolecular Medicine by Roger Williams and Dwight Kalita (Pergamon)
Clinical Ecology edited by Lawrence Dickey (Charles C. Thomas)

HYPOGLYCAEMIA

Body, Mind and Sugar by Dr E.M. Abrahamson and A.W. Pezet (Pyramid)
Is Low Blood Sugar Making You a Nutritional Cripple? by Ruth Adams and Frank Murray (Larchmont)
Low Blood Sugar by Martin L. Budd (Thorsons)

NUTRITION

Meganutrients and Your Nerves by Dr H. Newbold (Berkeley)
Let's Eat Right to Keep Fit by Adelle Davis (Allen & Unwin)
Let's Get Well by Adelle Davis (Allen & Unwin)
The Complete Carbohydrate Counter by Katie Stewart (Pan)

The Vitamin Bible by Earl Mindell (Arlington)
Your Vitamin Profile by Michael Colgan (Blond and Briggs)
   The last is highly recommended; quite simply the best on the market.

MISCELLANEOUS

The Stress of Life by Hans Selye (McGraw-Hill)
Silent Spring by Rachel Carson (Penguin)
The Yeast Connection by Dr. William Cook (Professional Books)

5 The Causative Role of the Thrush Organism in Multiple Allergies

Most people are used to thinking of thrush as a harmless, if annoying, condition that causes whitish plaques in babies' mouths and womens' genitals. Although it can be so unpleasant and profuse as to be debilitating, thrush as such is probably no more than this. But what has only recently become clear is what a sinister organism the thrush germ is: it appears to underlie a vast array of human ills and misery. A great many individuals have their lives ruined or made wretched by this organism without actually having thrush or realising it is the cause; in fact, very few doctors are aware of this new aspect to general health problems either.

The causative agent is a symbiotic yeast-like micro-organism called *Candida albicans*. It is a close relative of moulds that grow on stale food, and slightly more distant family members include mushrooms and cheeses. All of us are 'infected' by it shortly after birth; this is unavoidable since it is ubiquitous, living under nails, in the mouth, on the skin and in the intestines of an infant's immediate contacts. Fortunately for most of us, the presence of the organism does not signify overt, active disease; it is only when the host's defence mechanisms are lowered for any reason that it proliferates and takes over. Unless it reaches this stage, when thrush proper can be diagnosed by its clinical manifestations, doctors are accustomed to regarding it as a harmless commensal.

Unfortunately, it is not. Thanks largely to the pioneering work in the USA of Dr Orian Truss, an ecology-oriented psychiatrist, its role in a great deal of chronic illness has become known. The trouble is that although in most cases it coexists relatively innocently with human beings, if for any reason our immunity potential is lowered, as for example during prolonged periods of stress or illness, it gains the advantage. This enables the organism to grow in numbers, and can cause symptoms in a variety of ways. To begin with, it is allergenic: that is, it can provoke reactions leading to any of the enormous variety of symptoms that allergies are known to be capable of causing. Secondly, it seems to pave the way for absorption of many toxic substances from the bowel. *Candida* apparently infests the mucous lining of the gut to such an extent that its normal integrity breaks down and harmful foreign substances are allowed to pass from the lumen into the bloodstream. The effects of this vary enormously, but patients commonly experience mood changes: depression, anxiety, loss of memory and a number of other 'minor' mental symptoms. In exceptional cases, this can be more severe and lead to frightening conditions such as hallucination and even schizophrenia-like attacks.

The organism then becomes difficult to get rid of, even when the stress has passed. This is because it gains access to the *inside* of our body cells, and from there it cannot be dislodged: in other words it invades, and normal antibody defences will not function in this situation. What is of particular interest to readers of this book is that *Candida* has been shown unequivocally to *cause* multiple food and other allergies: its proper treatment and eradication can be crucial in terms of overcoming the allergy diathesis.

SYMPTOMS

An overgrowth of *Candida albicans* is a Fabian condition: it can lead to a bewildering variety of complaints which make it difficult to spot unless the practitioner has it uppermost in his or her mind. There is little doubt that these effects are created by more than one mechanism, as explained in the previous section; furthermore, individual reactions can change from day to day. Remembering what you read about 'target organs' earlier in the book, you will understand why this is so. Thus symptoms can be every bit as bizarre and irregular as those due to hidden allergies; plus there is the extra factor of toxicity caused by the infection.

You can imagine therefore that this peculiar illness has been very difficult to track down. Even now it is not fully understood, but considerable success in treating it leads us to believe that there has been a great advance in therapeutics. Almost all symptoms listed in the self-inventory (Chapter 4) can be caused by *Candida* overgrowth; thus it can at times be difficult – indeed, impossible – to dissociate its effects from those of allergy proper. The table in this appendix lists the symptoms or factors which are especially suggestive of trouble with this organism.

PATIENT HISTORY

Certain individuals are very prone to being invaded by the *Candida* organism, those who are already chronically sick being prime targets. In such cases the body's defences are already weakened and less able to repel attacks.

There is conclusive evidence that the frequent or long-term use of antibiotics causes a predisposition to the overgrowth of *Candida*. Broad-spectrum antibiotics especially, such as tetracycline and ampicillin (Penbritin), so beloved of the family GP, are responsible for starting off many invasions. The reason for this is that our own intestinal natural germs are one of the best defences against infection by 'wild' or foreign bugs. Large quantities of them live inside us and help in the breakdown of food and even in the manufacture of vitamins: we need them. When a doctor administers an antibiotic to treat sore throats (most of which are viral anyway, so the drug is useless) it kills these 'friendly' germs too. That leaves the way clear for something much worse to take over. Continuous antibiotics for a period of two months or more, or their frequent administration, say over four times in any one year, can be enough to set the stage for lifelong battles with *Candida*.

Use of the contraceptive pill is also known to be a predisposing factor. The enormous increase in *Candida* infections over the last twenty years in women of childbearing age is doubtless due to this cause.

Lastly, the causative role of poor diet, especially a preponderance of junk food, cannot be over-emphasised. If the body is not provided with adequate ammunition, it cannot fight.

Of course, if *Candida* infection has already been diagnosed, there can be no doubt about its success in overcoming body defences. Usually these attacks are recurring and very troublesome. One course of treatment may work, but the organism is soon back and before long treatment ceases to have any obvious benefit.

OVERCOMING THE PROBLEM

If you believe you might be a *Candida* victim, what should you do? It would be simple to say 'Consult your own doctor', but unfortunately at present few of them understand how to deal effectively with it; the most you are likely to get is a further course of treatment using drugs, which is unlikely to help in the long term. However, it may be an opportunity to get your condition properly diagnosed if you suffer from a vaginal discharge or similar affliction. This diagnosis is usually performed by taking samples and growing the organism on a culture medium. This will at least confirm your suspicions. If you have not been treated previously, there is certainly no reason not to agree to a course of tablets, pessaries or whatever is suggested.

If you have been harbouring thrush for a long time you may need more expert help. Practitioners who take an interest in medical alternatives and new work are comparatively rare, but they do exist. Action Against Allergy (Appendix 3) may be able to help by putting you in touch with such a person. It is possible to help yourself in overcoming the problem, and I give you some information here that may be of use. Unfortunately, treatment at present is not universally successful. It is important to realise tht we are up against a very tough opponent. Our counter-attack falls into several stages:

1 Preventative It is unwise to administer long-term antibiotics for trivial conditions such as acne or repeated sore throats. The pill is being implicated in more and more pathology; social factors aside, there is no *medical* justification for this form of contraception. As for an improvement in national eating habits, this is a major concern for forward-thinking doctors but rather beyond the scope of this monograph.

2 Eradicating the organism Traditional treatment using anti-fungal drugs (such as Nystan and Canesten) is most unsatisfactory: a typical short-term course rarely results in more than a temporary truce. It is the least important aspect of the campaign. Some clinical ecologists, however, have reported striking success using long-term (six months or more) treatment with powdered nystatin, a specific anti-*Candida* agent.

A diet higher than normal in fibre may help, since bulky stools give off fewer toxins and are voided quicker. Oat bran is suggested, but wheat bran is probably not a good choice, since wheat is a very common allergen.

3 Increasing body defences Helping the body to fight its own fight is by far the most promising approach. A good general diet concentrating on meat, fish, fruit and vegetables helps. These are less toxic foods than grains, sugar, dairy produce, stimulant drinks (tea and coffee) or manufactured 'fast foods' (junk).

Nutritional supplements are valuable, but care is required: for example, yeast derivatives such as vitamin B complex or brewer's yeast tablets, should be avoided. *Lactobacillus acidophilus* is an excellent dietary additive. It re-colonises the bowel and is effective in reducing the overgrowth of all foreign organisms, including *Candida*. It can be taken as a powder in a handy capsule form. Specific supplements would include:

Zinc (30-50 mg daily)
Vitamin A (10,000-20,000 IU daily)
Vitamin E (400-600 IU daily)
Vitamin C (2-4 g daily)
Pantothenic acid 500-1000 mg daily)

During the early phase of treatment, when inflammation and symptoms can still be quite severe, some workers suggest one copper aspirinate tablet daily. This should not be continued for longer than two or three weeks.

Finally, it should be pointed out that all of the above measures are relevant to remaining well once the problem has been overcome. Remember, *Candida* is still present: it merely stays quiescent.

TABLE OF SYMPTOMS ATTRIBUTABLE TO CANDIDA OVERGROWTH

Symptoms which are very positive factors:

Taken antibiotics for two months or longer
Persistent vaginal problems
Taken the pill for longer than two years
Symptoms worse in damp or mouldy places
Symptoms worse in damp weather
Taken any steroid drug for more than a month

Have persistent athlete's foot, crutch rash or ringworm
Headache or feeling unwell due to alcohol
Multiple food and chemical intolerances
Thrush already diagnosed and persistent

Symptoms which are suggestive:

Craving sugary or starchy foods
Craving alcohol
Fatigue, lethargy or 'feeling drained'
Abdominal pain or bloating
Diarrhoea or constipation
Aching joints
Aching and/or weak muscles

Premenstrual tension
Loss of sexual feeling, impotence
Headache
Poor memory
Mental confusion
Depression
Irritability
Frequent mood swings

Feeling unreal or depersonalised   Spots before the eyes
Vaginal itching, with or without   Endometriosis
   discharge   Numbness, burning or tingling
Dysmenorrhoea   sensations

Allergy sufferers will of course recognise many of these symptoms as
being identical to ones caused by allergies. *It is important to
understand that any of these symptoms may have other causes;
however, the more of these factors apply, the more certain it is that
Candida is the cause of your problem.*

6   Vitamin and Mineral Supplements

Until recently, the whole emphasis on sound nutrition was from the
point of view of supplementation. What was missing from the patient's
diet that resulted in disease?

   Now that the facts about food allergies are known, there has been a
shift: we now attach more importance to substances present in the diet
which shouldn't be rather than to what is missing. Nevertheless
deficiencies do occur, and they are significant. Vitamins and minerals
available and in the correct balance are essential to optimum health.
This in turn will affect the body's ability to cope with stressful
influences such as maladapted foods and chemicals; in other words,
these vital nutrients are part of the battle against allergies.

   Forget the myth of the average 'balanced diet' – it is misleading.
Modern research into nutrition makes such a concept as viable as the
flat earth theory. The usual quoted recommended daily allowances
(RDAs) are out of date and certainly inaccurate. RDAs also overlook
one significant point; a tremendous range of biological variation exists
from one individual to the next. This is true of many parameters,
including that of nutrition. To say we all need the same daily intake of
nutrients is as absurd as saying everyone is five feet two inches tall – it
simply isn't true!

   There are, moreover, other factors which should be taken into
account. Just because your diet has, in theory, all the right ingredients
is no assurance against deficiency: you may not be utilising all your
intake. We know very little about what influences there are on the
absorption of vitamins and minerals from the bowel. It is quite certain
that a large proportion of these substances escapes in the faeces. This

is particularly true of food allergy patients, many of whom have damaged or malfunctioning intestinal mucosa. An extreme of this is Coeliac 'disease', which is caused by intolerance of the protein gluten; victims suffer severe malnutrition due to the poor condition of the gut lining.

Furthermore, your food may not contain expected nutrient levels. The average orange may supposedly be rich in vitamin C, but Michael Colgan, author of *Your Vitamin Profile* (see Appendix 4), reports on testing typical oranges from a local supermarket and in some cases finding a *zero* vitamin level. The loss in this case would be due to storage and general deterioration. I have already explained that zinc deficiency is becoming common, since this mineral is now lacking even in the soil. Manufacturing reduces the nutritional content of most foods, often to almost nil. Disregard claims about 'added vitamins': the quantities put back are insignificant compared to those removed. The fact is that modern diets are a very poor index of nutritional status, except for the purpose of stating that some are wholly inadequate.

Finally, and most importantly, at times of stress your vitamin needs can sky-rocket: fifty or a hundred times the RDAs may be mopped up by the body and disappear into the system. Excesses are usually excreted, and this can be taken to be good presumptive evidence of the fact that these extra amounts are being utilised. Linus Pauling, one of the great men of our age, has lived to see vindicated his theory that vitamin C is a powerful anti-toxicity factor utilised in huge amounts by a body under siege from stressful influences, such as bacterial poisons in septicaemia.

WHAT THIS MEANS FOR YOU

As I have explained, allergy sufferers are often particularly at risk of vitamin and mineral deficiencies, due to their having damaged intestinal mucosa. This means that supplementation is even more important for you than for the rest of us. Major shortages may take many months or years to put right, even by the taking of quite large doses, so it is sensible to make a start as soon as possible.

In practice this means when you have almost completed the plan. It is no use taking huge amounts of pills only to find you have been making yourself mysteriously ill. Find out what your allergies are first; then experiment with supplements. And don't forget it is quite possible to be allergic to vitamin tablets. Be alert to the possibility and you are unlikely to come unstuck.

Try if you can to get preparations low in allergy potential. Some companies make special brands low in cereal, sugar and additives,

True-Free by Cantassium being an example. Avoid all tablets that are shiny or brightly coloured; in general, choose preparations which look and smell rather like stale grass – these are usually fairly natural.

MEGAVITAMINS VERSUS ORTHOMOLECULAR

These are two words which you will hear with increasing frequency as you delve into the world of nutrition. Basically, meganutrient therapy is based on the idea that if you give huge doses of everything there will be an abundance and that therefore shortages will be most unlikely. Most vitamins are not toxic, even in enormous doses, so little harm can be done. Even so-called toxic vitamins, such as vitamin A, are safe in large doses over a short period. The main objection is cost. Meganutrient therapy is rather like buying five motor cars just to be sure of having one which will start in the morning: by studying the problems of cold engines, you could save yourself a great deal of money!

Orthomolecular medicine, on the other hand, tries to estimate the exact needs of any given individual. Clearly, it won't be the same programme as for any other person, but general guidelines are applicable. Even the amounts recommended in orthomolecular prescribing exceed the RDAs by considerable margins. The tables I have prepared below would be in keeping with orthomolecular rather than meganutrient quantities. Both methods, of course, have their proponents. I suggest you read as widely as you can on the topic and make up your own mind.

SUGGESTED FORMULAS

These are suggestions for guidance only. It is not essential that you follow them blindly; nor are they likely to suit everyone. You may be better to take more or less than the stated doses. However, it is not advised that you get them too far out of step with one another: taking large amounts of one vitamin without taking the rest needed to act with it is largely a waste of time.

BASIC FORMULA

This is listed in two parts. Take one new tablet a day, and when you are successfully taking Step 1, then proceed to Step 2. If you have a reaction, ease off the dose or try a different preparation. For patients who are chronically short of vitamins (as for example in the case of those who have known many years of colitis), I often recommend they take the formulas anyway and be prepared to put up with symptoms, at least for the first few weeks. A good tip, if you should experience any ill effects after the doses, is to take all the pills last thing at night: with luck, you will sleep through the worst of the reaction!

Step 1

B1	50 mg
B2	50 mg
Niacin (B3)	500 mg
B6	100 mg
E	200 IU
A	10,000 IU
Magnesium	250 mg
Zinc	50 mg

Step 2

B12	20 mcg (or 2 capsules of dessicated liver)
Folic Acid	300 mcg
Choline	100 mg
PABA	50 mg
Inositol	100 mg
Biotin	300 mc
Vitamin D	200 IU
Iron (elemental iron)	20 mg
Manganese	5 mg
Selenium	25 mcg
Chromium	25 mcg
Iodine	50 mcg (or 2 tablets of kelp)
Lecithin	500 mcg

If you improve for a while on this regime and progress then tails off, it may be time to switch to a maintanance dose just to prevent any new deficiencies from developing. There are several multivitamin tablets available for this purpose. I usually recommend the vitamins and minerals made by the Cantassium Company for the Foresight Association. Similar products are Cantamega (again from Cantassium) or Multimax (from Nature's Best). Steer clear of firms involved in 'pyramid' health-produce selling; most of the money you spend goes on multi-level marketing, not on quality.

A number of good companies now produce vitamins free of unnecessary additives, such as sugar, corn and colourings. Check, when you buy, for these hypo-allergenic brands. If in any doubt, don't buy but shop elsewhere.

HAIR MINERAL ANALYSIS

For more information on your nutritional status, consider a hair
mineral analysis. Try Bio-Med International, 55 Queen's Road, East
Grinstead, Sussex RH19 1BG, cost £18, or in America Trace Analysis
Laboratories, PO Box 4235, Heyward, California 94540, USA.

A hair analysis can reveal a great deal of useful information about
the levels of minerals in your body. However, it must be said that the
help of a physician skilled in interpretation is necessary to take full
advantage of the results – there are very few of us!

There are many excellent books on vitamins, and some downright
misleading ones. Remember, nutrition is still in its infancy and
developing rapidly; thus you may expect some conflicting information.
Don't let this confuse you. The fact is, the more you read the more you
will be able to make up your own mind. Don't leave it to a doctor:
nutrition is everyone's business, not just for 'experts'. See Appendix 4
for suggested books on the subject.

Index